The DIET ALTERNATIVE

P9-DHJ-173

The DIET ALTERNATIVE

DIANE HAMPTON

📧 *Whitaker House*

Unless otherwise indicated, all Scripture quotations are taken from the *King James Version* (KJV) of the Bible.

Scripture quotations marked (TLB) are from *The Living Bible*, © Tyndale House Publishers, Wheaton, Illinois, 1971 and used by permission.

THE DIET ALTERNATIVE

ISBN: 0-88368-148-X
Printed in the United States of America
Copyright © 1984 by Whitaker House

Whitaker House
580 Pittsburgh Street
Springdale, PA 15144

8 9 10 11 12 13 14 15 / 05 04 03 02 01 00 99 98 97 96

CONTENTS

While this book is specifically oriented to overeating, these same principles can be used to overcome *smoking*, *drinking*, and other areas of *compulsive behavior*. God wants us to walk in victory in every area of our life!

"If the Son therefore shall make you free, ye shall be free indeed"—John 8:36

Chapter 1

DELIVERANCE FROM GLUTTONY

I can still remember going to my personal physician some twelve or thirteen years ago. I was deeply involved in compulsive eating, and there was such a feeling of desperation watching my weight go up and up as it had so many times before. I knew that it was out of control, but I didn't know how to get that control back.

I remember explaining to my doctor what I was going through and how frightened I was. After listening to me for a few minutes, he left the room and came back with a 1000 calorie a day diet. How could he have had so little understanding! *If I could have stayed on a diet, I wouldn't have had a weight problem!* I knew how many calories there were in everything I ate. But knowing that still didn't stop me from overeating.

Desperate!

Once I gained thirty pounds in three months. Food was on my mind constantly. When I woke up in the morning, my first thoughts were about what I would eat that day. I wondered if I would be able to control my eating at all, or if I would succumb to my desire to gorge. Even when I was on one of my frequent diets (periodically I was able to regain my normal weight and keep it for a few months), I was obsessed with thoughts of food. I was also usually depressed.

I read every diet and weight control book I could find. I tried "self-hypnosis." I went to a physician for hypnosis. I went to a psychologist. I even went to a weight doctor. *But there was something inside me that continued to drive me to overeat.*

Experiencing Sin's Control

Paul knew what it was to be under the control of sin. If you substitute the words *eating* and *overeating* for *sin* in Paul's letter to the Romans, you have a good explanation of what it's like to be a compulsive eater. Even more important, you see what it takes to overcome it.

"I don't understand myself at all, for I really want to do (eat) what is right, but I can't. I do (eat) what I don't want to—what I hate (a person will eat almost anything on a binge). *I know perfectly well that what I am doing (eating) is wrong, and my bad conscience proves that I agree with these laws I am breaking* (condemnation is a constant companion of a compulsive eater). *But I can't help myself, because I'm no*

longer doing it. It is sin inside me that is stronger than I am that makes me do these evil things (this overeating).

"I know I am rotten through and through so far as my old sinful nature is concerned. No matter which way I turn I can't make myself do right (eat right) (psychology, hypnosis, crash diets). *I want to but I can't. When I want to do good (try to diet) I don't (eat anyway); and when I try not to do wrong (eat), I do it anyway. Now if I am doing what I don't want to, it is plain where the trouble is: sin still has me in it's evil grasp"* (Romans 7:15-20 *TLB*).

"Oh, what a terrible predicament I'm in! Who will free me from my slavery to this deadly overeating?"

How You Can Be Free

"Thank God! Jesus Christ our Lord did it! He has set me free!" *"So there is now no condemnation awaiting those who belong to Christ Jesus. For the power of the life-giving Spirit—and this power is mine through Christ Jesus—has freed me from the vicious circle of sin and death (overeating and guilt). We aren't saved from sin's grasp by knowing the commandments of God (how to diet), because we can't and don't keep them, but God put into effect a different plan to save us. He sent his own Son in a human body like ours—except that ours are sinful— and destroyed sin's (overeating's) control over*

11

us by giving Himself as a sacrifice for our sins (overeating). So now we can obey God's laws (overcome overeating) if we follow after the Holy Spirit and no longer obey the old evil nature within us.

"Those who let themselves be controlled by their lower natures (overeating, sowing to the flesh) *live only to please themselves, but those who follow after the Holy Spirit find themselves doing those things that please God"* (Romans 8:1-5 *TLB*). The victory is there, but we must choose to receive it.

I remember, as a compulsive eater, looking at people who never had a weight problem. I could not even imagine what it felt like to not be concerned with and controlled by food. I remember reading an article about Johnny Carson where he made a statement about not really caring what he ate.

He said he ate because it was something he had to do. It was impossible for me to relate to that statement. I remember thinking what a strange remark that was and wondering if that was how it felt to be in control of your eating.

Living In Control

Now after being completely healed for over ten years, I know what control feels like. Sometimes it is hard for me to remember what it was like as a glutton because God put my sins as far "as the east is from the west, so far hath he removed our transgressions from us" (Psalm 103:12).

Today I can think of hundreds of things I would rather do than eat. I often get busy during the day and realize about 4:00 p.m. that I haven't eaten all day. Then I get a real hunger response from my body. I enjoy food much more now because there is no condemnation when I eat. It is amazing how much better food tastes when you are genuinely hungry.

One thing I really enjoy is throwing out leftover cake or pie. I guess you have to have been a compulsive eater to really appreciate this experience. In the past, these things would have always been eaten, often in one day! Right now we are eating a box of chocolates that was given to us a month ago.

Now that is freedom!

Jesus said, *"If the Son therefore shall make you free, ye shall be free indeed"* (John 8:36). I now have freedom to have one chocolate instead of half a box or two or three chocolate chip cookies instead of a dozen. I am free indeed!

The Source Of My Release

Another new and wonderful experience is not changing dress sizes. At every change of season, I had clothes I could not wear. They were either too big or too small because my size was constantly changing. I haven't changed dress sizes in ten years, and I have had two children during those ten years. It will work for you, too, for the rest of your life.

I'll never stop thanking God for sending Jesus to save me from this gluttony and depression. The joy does not subside but *"is like the shining light, that shineth more and more unto the perfect day"* (Proverbs 4:18). There is no more darkness inside of me, no more hidden part.

I remember, when I had been binging and someone came to the door, the feeling of not wanting to be with other people. I felt as if they somehow knew I had been eating too much. There was always that hidden part of me, that sin and darkness, that only I knew about.

When I was born again, it was as though a light came on inside me. That light was Jesus Christ and He overcame the darkness. The sensation of light is so real inside me now that sometimes I think I could glow in the dark! We do glow in the dark in a sense. Our light shines forth in a dark world. We are the light of the world.

All Things Are New

I was born again late one night when I was all alone. In my church we repeated a creed which said in part, *"I believe in one God, the Father Almighty, Maker of Heaven and earth. . .and in one Lord Jesus Christ, the only begotten Son of God."*

When you truly realize who Jesus is and what He did for us, your whole life can be changed. *"Old things are passed away; behold, all things are become new"* (2 Corinthians 5:17). Scriptures which I heard almost all of my life became real to me. Jesus became the Lord of my life. His death and resurrection, which saved me from my sins, became exciting to me because it was *personal!* Jesus died for *me!* I found a Source for my life, a Teacher, a Word that was Truth itself and would never change or let me down. I found a place to take this sin which had been inside me.

A New Life

I am thankful that the weight did not just drop off because someone laid hands on me, although I thank God for the supernatural in our lives. I didn't just lose weight; I found a new way of life! I learned that Jesus is truly *"able to keep (me) from falling, and to present (me) faultless before the presence of his glory with exceeding joy"* (Jude 24). I learned that God's Word is true, and I learned how to apply it to my life and receive healing. Because of this, *I* have found "exceeding joy that does not diminish."

The Lord is more real to me today than He was that night ten years ago. He continues to be my Savior.

As long as we live on this earth, *Satan will never stop trying to gain a foothold in our lives, but Jesus will never stop being our Savior from that sin.* Salvation never stops being a choice, but as long as we choose Jesus, sin will have no power over us.

Gluttony is a spiritual problem. Until that "spirit of overeating" is gone, you will never live in lasting victory over your weight. Conversely, once it is gone, eating will never again be a problem in your life.

Chapter 2

NOT HAVING SPOT, WRINKLE, OR STRETCHMARK

Overeating is a spiritual problem, and it has a spiritual solution. In our classes, we call this thing inside us that makes us want to overeat "the spirit of overeating." The Bible calls it gluttony. This spirit of overeating is like a living thing inside a person. Eventually, it can grow until it controls our lives. It can become a stronghold.

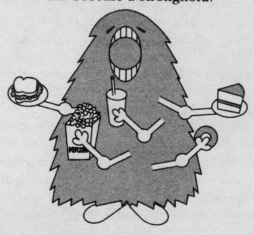

Did you ever notice that when Scripture mentions a glutton, it also mentions a drunkard? That is because the same spirit which causes a person to drink too much also causes a person to eat too much. A glutton is no more in control of his eating than a drunkard is of his drinking. The drunkard says, "I could stop drinking if I really wanted to." The glutton says, "I could lose weight if I really wanted to." Yet, each knows the frightening truth that they are no longer in control.

Fighting Flesh

Paul tells us in 2 Corinthians 10:4, *"the weapons of our warfare are not carnal."* Every overweight person has experienced the frustration of fighting this spiritual battle with carnal or fleshly weapons. Dieting is a carnal weapon. Dieting starves your body, but it does not affect the spirit of overeating which is inside. That is why you can go on a diet and lose weight, then stop the diet and gain it all back. *Jesus never put a glutton on a diet.*

A person can be just as obsessed with food when he is on a diet as when he is overeating. He still thinks about food just as much.

There are some highly successful diet plans which allow you to eat a great deal of food, but only certain types. You can have some things in unlimited amounts such as carrot sticks and celery. Instead of eating potato chips and cookies, you munch on carrots and celery. Instead of eating

18

huge servings of baked beans and pota~~~~~~
eat huge servings of green beans and b~~~~~

It is like a heroin addict going on meth~~~~
the addiction is still there, but you take~~~~ ~~~~a-
done instead of the more destructive heroin. The
glutton continues in gluttony but eats low calorie
foods instead of high calorie foods. And, he loses
weight. *The urge to overeat is still there. The
habit of overeating is still there.*

When a person eventually grows tired of preparing special diet foods and considering everything
he must eat for the diet, he eventually goes back to
foods he ate before the diet. Because he has not
dealt with his gluttony, he regains the lost weight.
But Jesus said, "If the son therefore shall make you
free, *ye shall be free indeed!*" (John 8:36).

Freedom From Restrictions

Being free means not having to bring special
food with you to a restaurant. Being free is not
spending half of your day planning menus. Being
free is not cooking one meal for your family and a
separate meal for yourself. Being free is not having
to pass up half of the food your hostess serves.
Being free is being free indeed.

When you are on a diet, you lose weight. When
you stop the diet, you regain the weight. It's like a
roller coaster, with each period of gaining more
discouraging than the last. Some people eventually give up. Their weight increases, out of con-

., leading to many serious health complications.

An overweight person is more likely to develop high blood pressure, heart disease, diabetes, breast cancer, arterial disease, pregnancy complications, and less likely to survive surgery. Their very life expectancy is shortened.

Conversely, grossly overweight people sometimes diet to the point of starvation. They severely restrict their eating and continue to diet, even when they have lost weight, to the point of becoming seriously underweight. This condition, called "anorexia nervosa," is fatal in many cases because the spiritual weakness has not been dealt with. The eating is still out of control. Satan's ultimate purpose is always the same, *"to steal, and to kill and to destroy"* (John 10:10).

Power For Freedom

A compulsive eater must realize, from God's Word, that *gluttony is sin.* This is not to bring them under condemnation but rather *to a conviction of the Holy Spirit with repentance and freedom.* Condemnation brings on more eating. But conviction brings repentance, and repentance brings the *power* of God into our lives. That power brings *freedom.* You will never be free as long as you keep excusing yourself by saying, "It doesn't really matter." God's Word says that it does matter!

Proverbs 23:21 tells us that the *"drunkard and*

the glutton shall come to poverty." Again in Proverbs 23:2, *"put a knife to the throat, if thou be a man given to appetite"* (put the sword of God's Word to thy throat if thou be a man given to appetite). In Philippians 3:18-19, Paul tells us, *"For many walk, of whom I have told you often, and now tell you even weeping that they are the enemies of the cross of Christ: whose end is destruction, whose God is their belly."* Without repentance, there can be no freedom from sin.

We would be quick to deal with a church full of drunkards, but we are afraid to "hurt someone's feelings" if they are a glutton. Let me tell you from experience, *they are hurting already, more than you can imagine.*

One of the women in our class who has been a special blessing to me gave her testimony. She said that, when she sought help in her church, people told her that size "didn't really matter," even though she weighed over 350 pounds! Her body was literally being destroyed, her soul and spirit were in condemnation, and Christians told her "it doesn't really matter."

Conviction vs. Condemnation

I don't believe I have ever heard a person tell a drunk "it really doesn't matter" how much they drink. But how often have we told a glutton that it doesn't really matter? "We love you just the way you are." *God's Word says it does matter. God's*

21

Word says there is freedom from all unrighteousness for the believer.

Loving a glutton has never been a problem. In fact, it's very non-threatening having a fat friend. It's a question of the glutton loving himself. It's a question of living in victory. Jesus tells us to *"be ye therefore perfect, even as your Father which is in heaven is perfect"* (Matthew 5:48). Literally destroying your body with excess fat or constant weight changes is not being perfect. God always loves us, but He wants things better for us.

Sin does not offend God simply because He is holy; it offends Him because it is contrary to the way we were created. God hates sin because He knows it destroys us.

A drunk can become obnoxious, disruptive, or abusive. A glutton seldom is. He is often a person with a gentle disposition and a tender heart. *But he is hurting inside just as much, he is hurting his body just as much, and he needs ministering just as much.* A drunk does not hesitate to ask for counseling, help, or prayer; but where does a glutton go? Most people look the other way or tell their children not to say anything about how fat so-and-so is. We even bring them candy or fix their favorite foods.

In our Scriptural Eating Classes, we have a questionnaire we ask each person to complete. One of the questions is, "Do you believe that it is sinful to overeat?" The unanimous answer is, *"Yes."* The response often stems from condemnation, not

Holy Spirit conviction. I was desperately aware that I was "rotten through and through" as Paul puts it in Romans 7:18 (Living Bible), but I didn't know how to get out of it. Gluttons need to know that they are holy through and through—that Jesus died that they might be *free from gluttony*.

Origins Of Gluttony

Gluttony comes from Satan. To overcome it we need to have the *"eyes of* (our) *understanding being enlightened; that* (we) *may know what is the hope of* (our) *calling, and what the riches of the glory of* (our) *inheritance in the saints* (with regard to gluttony) *and what is the exceeding greatness of his power to us-ward who believe,* (with regard to gluttony) *according to the working of his mighty power"* (Ephesians 1:18-19).

There is no reason for any "born-again" believer to have an eating problem ever again. We are told that Christ is coming after a "Glorious church, not having spot, or wrinkle"—or stretchmark! (Ephesians 5:27).

Chapter 3

SEEDS OF GLUTTONY

People often ask me, "Diane, when did you *know* you were truly healed of gluttony?" I have to answer honestly that, for the whole first year, I had to keep pinching myself to believe it was going to last. After many years of frustration, disappointment, and dead-end diets, I knew it would take a miracle to set me free!

I did not thoroughly understand that I could be completely healed of gluttony and free for the rest of my life. I was hoping for the ability to keep my eating under control. But, *"eye hath not seen, nor ear heard, neither have entered into the heart of man, the things which God hath prepared for them that love Him"* (1 Corinthians 2:9).

Many times I dreamed I would be thin, free, and "normal." Yet, I always woke up to the same driving desire to eat. I had a constant obsession with food. Now, for the first time, it was gone—not under control—but gone! Depression and self-hatred were lifted from me as giant weights never to return. After years and years of constant weight changes, I had the extraordinary experience of being able to wear the same clothes year after year. Every change of season was a new reminder that I was free!

Help For Your Problem

We have a twelve-year old daughter who is very creative and extremely sensitive. Sometimes life seems to overwhelm her. At times like this I hold her in my arms, pat her back, and tell her, "It's going to be all right. Everything is going to be OK. You are going to have a wonderful life." Sometimes she comes to me and says, "Mom, would you hug me and tell me everything's going to be all right?"

For all of you who have struggled so long and hard with compulsive eating, you who feel discouraged and overwhelmed, if Jesus could be there with you, I know He would do the same for you. He would wrap His arms around you and tell you, "It's going to be all right. I can help you. I know the answer, and you can be free."

How Does Gluttony Begin?

To understand the solution, we need to have some understanding of how gluttony begins in a life, how it becomes a stronghold. We have a number of Scriptural examples of Jesus feeding our physical bodies. There was always a consistent order. First, spirits were fed and then bodies were fed. First, He taught and ministered to the spirit, then He multiplied the loaves and fishes to feed the body.

"And they say unto him, we have here but five loaves, and two fishes. He said, Bring them hither to me. And he commanded the multitude to sit down on the grass, and took the five loaves, and the two fishes, and looking up to heaven, he blessed, and brake, and gave the loaves to his disciples, and the disciples to the multitude. And they did all eat, and were filled: and they took up the fragments that remained twelve baskets full" (Matthew 14:17-20).

Gluttony begins when this system gets out of order. A person feels frustrated, bored, angry, or lonely, but rather than dealing with the spiritual problem, they eat. These are the "deceitful meats" spoken of in Proverbs 23:2. It is food eaten for the wrong reason—to avoid dealing with the deeper problem.

Loving Jesus First

Jesus gave us one great commandment, *"Thou shalt love the Lord thy God with all thy heart, and with all thy soul, and with all thy mind, and with all thy strength: this is the first commandment"* (Mark 12:30). In gluttony, rather than loving God with the whole mind, a person begins to eat when he is bored or worried. Rather than loving God with all his soul, a person begins to eat when he is frustrated or angry. Rather than loving

God with all his heart, he begins to eat when he is lonely, depressed, or defeated. That is why Paul said in Phillipians 3:19 that a glutton's *"god is their belly."*

Spiritual Seed

When we eat this way, the seeds of gluttony are sown. We are told in Galatians 6:7: *"be not deceived: God is not mocked; for whatsoever a man soweth, that shall he also reap. For he that soweth to his flesh* (eating for the wrong reasons) *shall of the flesh reap corruption* (gluttony); *but he that soweth to the Spirit* (seeking help in God's Word) *shall of the Spirit reap life everlasting* (Spirit controlled life)."

A person who has never eaten out of frustration, anger, boredom, or loneliness finds it hard to imagine why a person would do this. But, *as with all sin, in the beginning he finds real pleasure in overeating.* As a drunk drinks himself into a stupor, a glutton eats himself into a stupor. The food tastes good and seems to help him forget about his problems. Unfortunately, as with all sin, when the pleasure begins to wear off, the addictive quality of sin does not. Jesus warns us, *"Whosoever committeth sin is the servant of sin"* (John 8:34).

Seeking Solace In Wrong Places

The basic problems which caused the person to seek solace in food in the first place have not been dealt with. As a result, the problems are only

27

increased. More often than not, depression accompanies gluttony. The original frustration is accompanied by even greater frustration as the eating gets out of control. The original anger is accompanied by condemnation and greater anger at oneself. "I hate myself when I overeat like this" is a common response.

Tears of anger, frustration, and hopelessness accompany each binge. It is not unlike drug addiction in that the "highs" become less high, and the "lows" become more and more unbearable. Proverbs says, "Bread of deceit is sweet to a man; but afterward his mouth shall be filled with gravel" (Proverbs 20:17).

The Solution

Because gluttony begins in the spirit, the solution also begins in the spirit. It began by sowing to the flesh, and it will end by sowing to the Spirit!

In the past I had sown "to the flesh" by eating during my times of depression, frustration, boredom, and guilt. Now I began to sow "to the Spirit" by fasting and filling myself with God's Word.

Every glutton has experienced the "supernatural" (demonic) urge to overeat, even eating things they don't really like. Proverbs 27:7 tells us that to the full soul, even a honeycomb isn't tempting, "but to the hungry soul, every bitter thing is sweet." God's Word is also supernatural and can fill that hungry soul. As I began to sow to the

Spirit, I began to experience a supernatural desire not to overeat.

The condemnation that Satan heaped on me was losing its power over me. That urge to eat to my destruction began to subside.

First comes the inner healing, then comes the outer healing which is the weight loss. After the inner healing, *that awful, constant, nagging urge to overeat is gone.* When I dieted as a glutton, I was confronted with temptation from the moment I woke up in the morning. I didn't have to stand against eating a few times a day; I had to stand against eating every 15 minutes! Cutting back on eating is such a simple thing now.

Where To Begin

In Matthew 17:20-21, Jesus tells us, *"If ye have faith as a grain of mustard seed, ye shall say unto this mountain, Remove hence to yonder place; and it shall remove; and nothing shall be impossible unto you. Howbeit this kind goeth not out but by prayer and fasting."* Gluttony is one of these things. There is sometimes a lifetime pattern of overeating which must be broken. Eating carrot sticks and celery, instead of potato chips and cookies, does not break this pattern.

No one became a glutton or compulsive eater in one day. Gluttony becomes a stronghold because, as Jesus said, *"Whosoever committeth sin is the servant of sin"* (John 8:34). It did not begin as a stronghold. It began as a small seed, and it began to grow when we first began to "sow to the flesh" by eating from frustration, loneliness, anger, self-condemnation, and habit.

Each time we used food this way, this urge to indulge grew a little bigger and a little stronger. Gluttony consists of two forces. One is an overwhelming desire to eat with constant, nagging thoughts of food. This is the spiritual part which we call the "spirit of overeating." The other part is simply habit. A compulsive eater often gets to the point where he or she is actually unaware of some of the food they eat. Overeating has become as natural as breathing.

Hidden Sin

One woman in class shared how God showed her that she always scooped a heaping spoonful of peanut butter for herself when she made her children peanut butter sandwiches. She said she was honestly unaware of eating the peanut butter.

Eventually gluttony, or the "spirit of overeating," becomes like a strong, healthy, living plant inside us. It is a stronghold, a fortified place surrounded by excuses, self-deception, and habits which can be formed over a lifetime. Each time we choose God over our eating, we chip away another root of the stronghold.

Gluttony is like a huge tree which can be blown over by a mild wind when the root structure is destroyed. The spirit of overeating shrivels up a little more with each victory until it finally dies.

Gluttony begins with sowing to the flesh. It will end by sowing to the Spirit, in faith.

Daily Fasting

God's Word says, *"Whatsoever a man soweth, that shall he also reap. For he that soweth to his flesh* (eating out of frustration, boredom, anger, or other reasons) *shall of the flesh reap corruption* (gluttony, compulsive eating, obsession with food); *but he that soweth to the Spirit* (daily periods of fasting) *shall of the Spirit reap life everlasting* (a Spirit-controlled life)" (Galatians 6:7-9).

Jesus said that when we fast we are to *"Fast. . .unto thy Father which is in secret: and thy Father, which seeth in secret, shall reward thee openly."* (Matthew 6:16,18). He did not say, *"If* ye fast," but rather *"when* ye fast." If you need control with your eating, you must sow "control with your eating." As you do, *release your faith to God.*

This type of fasting attacks gluttony at both levels. Releasing your faith to God as you sow control attacks the spiritual force of gluttony. The physical side of fasting helps to break the habit. There is a saying, "Sow an action and you reap a habit."

Fasting Before God

My approach to weight loss was always to "diet before men" rather than "fast in secret before God." My healing began when I literally applied this Scripture to my compulsive eating and released my faith to God for a miracle! During my healing, not even my husband knew I was fasting. My diets were always obvious—one meal for him, something else for me. Now I would eat breakfast and fast until dinner. When he came home, I ate regular meals with him, but smaller portions.

This fasting was not just another way of losing weight. It was a secret commitment between God and me. Every time I passed up some food, I released my faith to God for healing. This is where the *power* is. Jesus said, *"as many as received Him* (choose Him), *to them gave He power to become sons of God"* (John 1:12). We don't have to provide the power, just the will. To this day, I am not a person strong in will power, but I have learned the strength of leaning on the power of Jesus Christ.

Secrets To Effective Fasting

This fasting should not be a week-long fast or a three-day fast, but rather a daily period of fasting. Skipping one meal a day is an ideal and Scripturally sound way of fasting (see Chapter 4).

In the beginning your body will protest—*I'm going to starve without food because I missed a meal!!* Satan will try to pull you away from God's Word. He will try to tell you it isn't going to work. "You have always been overweight and you always will be overweight." He will try to get you to binge. But Scripture says, *"Resist the devil, and he will flee from you"* (James 4:7).

Purpose in your heart each morning which seed you are going to sow. Don't wait until lunchtime to decide you are going to fast lunch! One woman said she purposed to fast until noon. At noon she found she could go longer, so she determined to go until 2:00 p.m. At 2:00 she found she could fast longer, so she decided to fast until dinner. And she did.

Proverb 3:3 talks about writing on the "table of (our) heart." I found that if I resolved to fast a certain time before the Lord, I never failed. If I only thought "maybe I will sow some fasting today," I usually failed.

Does God Mean More To You?

When I am fasting before God, and I am tempted to eat, I simply ask myself, "Which means more to me? This food or Jesus?" Looking at food this way makes it easy for me to choose. I love the Lord with all my heart, and all of a sudden that food doesn't mean much.

One exercise we sometimes do in our Scriptural Eating Classes is especially helpful when having a problem with particular foods such as chocolate. For me, gumdrops were an irresistible temptation.

We actually bring the various "problem foods" to class. Problem foods are any food in which we consistently overeat. Sometimes it is a food we don't normally consider a problem food, such as apples. You can sinfully overeat any food!

We take the food in our hands and, as we look at it, we make a decision that we love God more than we love that food. Then we pray together. "Lord, I love You more than this candy bar. I ask Your Holy Spirit to remind me that I love You more than this food every time I am tempted to overeat this week."

Anytime you are having a problem with a certain food, do this. As you pray over that food, decide you love God more than that food. All week that food will seem different to you because the Holy Spirit is helping you. I remember the first time I did this. Every time I saw that food, the Holy Spirit would call to mind my decision and the victory was quick!

Sowing Good Seed

In 2 Corinthians 9:6 we are told, *"He which soweth sparingly shall reap also sparingly; and he which soweth bountifully shall reap also bountifully."* What is frugal sowing and what is bountiful sowing with regard to our fasting? We are told, *"The Lord seeth not as a man seeth; for man looketh on the outward appearance, but the Lord looketh on the heart"* (1 Samuel 16:7). God is always looking at our heart.

Jesus was greatly moved by a certain type of giving. Remember the little widow that Jesus commended in Mark 12:44? It was because she "gave of her want" that Jesus commended her. He wasn't impressed with the rich people who "did cast in of their abundance," but oh, how He noticed the widow! How He felt her faith reach out to God as she gave "all that she had." Jesus was moved by this bountiful giving.

Contrast this with frugal giving. If you normally do not eat breakfast, then not eating breakfast is not "giving of your want." It is not bountiful giving, and it is not sowing from your heart.

Results Of Sparse Sowing

A woman in one class actually did this! She didn't seem to be having much success, yet she said, "I've been fasting a meal every day!" I asked her which meal she was fasting, and she said breakfast (the smallest meal). I asked her if she normally ate breakfast, since most overweight people don't.

"Well, no," was her reply. She sowed sparingly and was reaping sparingly! God knew she didn't eat breakfast! Even if she did, this would be the smallest and least significant meal to fast. He was looking for a heart response that said, "Lord, I love you more than this food." He was looking for a heart that soared in faith as it gave in joy! Instead, he found deception and avarice.

Jesus said in Mark 10:29 that it was only what we gave up "for *His sake* and the gospel's" that would be returned to us a hundredfold. God looks for our inner motivation.

Sowing Bountifully

If your boss tells you that you *must* work through your lunch hour, then not eating lunch is not sowing bountifully. If you gave up lunch because your boss said you *must*—it was not for the sake of Jesus. However, sometimes working through your lunch hour *is* bountiful giving. Perhaps you resolved in your heart that morning you were going to fast lunch. God might have arranged for your boss to ask you to work through your lunch hour to help you make it.

The Bible says that the *"steps of a just man are ordered of the Lord"* (Psalm 37:23). Expect God to get involved when you sow in faith! Many times when I decided to fast, God brought activities into my day which made it almost impossible to find time to eat. He made it easy for me.

It is the motivation of our heart and giving in faith that determines bountiful giving. Sometimes not eating one cookie is bountiful giving! God sees that one cookie the same way He saw the widow's mite.

If you have the most trouble with overeating at bedtime, this is the time you should fast before God. This would be seeding from your want. If you have trouble because you eat while fixing dinner for your family, this is the time you should fast before God. If you do not eat all the time, but eat too much when you do eat, begin by cutting out second helpings and offering the sacrifice to God.

Whenever you are overeating is the time to sow from your want. That is loving God with all your strength in regard to eating.

One Day At A Time

Jesus told us to take one day at a time. *"Take therefore no thought for the morrow: for the morrow shall take thought for the things of itself. Sufficient unto the day is the evil thereof"* (Matthew 6:34). Jesus is telling us not to try to handle the whole problem at once. We have enough grace to walk in total victory for each day, but if we focus on the 100 or 50 pounds we have to lose, we aren't going to reach our goal.

I remember getting up in the morning and weighing myself. Seeing how much weight I needed to lose was such a discouragement that, instead of beginning small, I thought about all the food I was going to have to do without. I would consider how long it would take and often I would give up before I began!

Humanly, we always look at the whole problem, and it seems impossible. But Jesus taught us to start small and have faith in God. Jesus said, *"the things which are impossible with men are possible with God"* (Luke 18:27).

We become like the fishermen in Luke, chapter 5 who were fishing all night. Jesus said, *"let down your nets for a draught."* The fishermen answered, *"Master, we have toiled all the night."* They were thinking that they had cast the net over and over, and it would be useless to cast the net one more time. We often think, "But I've tried every diet and nothing has worked. What good will it do to stop between meal eating or to try to change my activities?"

When they cast their nets at the word of Jesus, they caught more fish than they could handle! Jesus is also involved in *our* lives. We are not just fasting between meals, we are sowing our fast to God as a farmer sows seed. We are each watching eagerly for a harvest.

Faithful Living

I found that as I tried to be faithful for just that day for that hour, the weeks took care of themselves. How much emotional illness is a result of anxiety about the future or guilt over the past. God who created us tells us that we will overload the circuits! *"Sufficient unto this day is the evil thereof. Take no thought for the morrow"* (Matthew 6:34). Just try to make it this day.

Jesus told us, *"He who is faithful in that which is least*—daily periods of fasting—*will be faithful also in much*—total weight loss," (Luke 16:10). The more faithful I was in small decisions, the more faithful I was in the big ones.

Our Free Will Choice

No one can sow the seed but you. No one else can do it for you. The choice is yours. You never lose your free will as far as God is concerned. You can try to blame others for your choices. You may blame your husband. "He makes me so mad, I can't keep from eating!" You may blame your family. "I came from a fat family," or "Satan simply has me under his thumb with my eating." Or, your childhood eating habits may have been wrong. "I was raised to eat wrong."

God tells us the choice is ours. *"I have set before you life and death, blessing and cursing: therefore choose life"* (Deuteronomy 30:19). *"Know ye not that to whom ye yield yourselves servants* (whom you choose) *to obey, his servants ye are to whom ye obey; whether of sin unto death, or of obedience unto righteousness?"* (Romans 6:16). God will supply the power, but we must supply the will.

There was a time in my life when it was impossible for me to control my eating for any length of time. But, *"The things which are impossible with men are possible with God"* (Luke 18:27).

Chapter 4

HUNGRY AND FULL

"In the beginning God created the heaven and the earth. . . .And God said, let us make man in our image. . .And the Lord God planted a garden eastward in Eden; and there he put the man whom he had formed. . . .And the Lord God commanded the man, saying, Of every tree of the garden thou mayest freely eat. . .And God saw every thing that he had made, and, behold, it was very good" (Genesis 1:1,26; 2:8,16;1:31).

In this man whom God created, He put a response called "hunger." This response came when the man needed food. The system was very good. And God put another response in the man called "full." This response came when his body had enough food. It was also very good. These responses, hungry and full, calculated exactly how much food the man needed to eat, for he was *"fearfully and wonderfully made"* (Psalm 139:14).

Some foods were heavy, and this full response

came quickly and lasted a long time. Some foods were lighter, and the full response came more slowly. But no matter what was eaten—goats or grapes—these two responses were his guides for eating and not eating. There were no gluttons in the garden.

Recapturing Your Natural Responses

When a newborn baby is brought home from the hospital, he makes good use of these responses. He cries when he is hungry, and we feed him. When he is full he stops eating, and we stop trying to feed him. It all works very well—just as God intended. We are born with these responses so we don't have to learn them. Doctors have even given this a name. It is called "demand feeding." Babies eat when they are hungry and stop eating when they are full.

Unfortunately, this is usually the last we hear of these hungry and full responses. A child still responds to these God-given responses, and we see how well it works. One rarely sees an overweight child. But as he grows, we begin to give the child a cracker when he is bored or a cookie when he is tired. By the time the child is five years old, if he sits down to dinner and is not hungry, he is often told, "You can just sit right there until you clean your plate."

If the child cleans his plate, he is told he is a "good boy." If the child does not clean his plate, he is told he is "bad."

Reasons For Eating

We learn to eat because "it's time," "you feel better if you eat," "you *might* get hungry," "people are starving in India," or "you will hurt Aunt Mabel's feelings if you don't eat." These are all typical reasons for eating.

By adulthood these God-given responses of hungry and full have often been hidden so successfully that many count calories, carbohydrates, or whatever to determine how much food they need. *We never dream of skipping a meal just because we aren't hungry.* At best, we simply don't eat quite as much.

One of the first things God showed me about my eating was to *eat only when you are hungry.* Never stop any activity because it is "time to eat." "Time to eat" is when your body gives you a real hunger response. Everyone has experienced times when they were involved in something interesting or exciting and have inadvertently missed a meal. It was completely painless—they simply became involved in something interesting and forgot to eat.

Jesus had this effect on people. They often followed to hear Him teach with no thought about what they would eat. In Matthew 14, we are told how the people followed Him from the cities into the desert. He taught and healed their sick all day long. Before they knew it, it was evening, and they were out in the desert with nothing to eat! Five thousand men, women, and children who did not think about food all day long!

Deal With The Spiritual Then The Physical

Jesus was moved with compassion, multiplied the five loaves and two fishes, and fed the 5,000 people. They all ate until they were "filled." Notice the order of these events. *First,* He dealt with the spiritual—He taught and healed. *Then* and only then did He even think about food.

In Matthew 15 we see Jesus departing to a mountain by the Sea of Galilee. Great multitudes followed Him as He sat down to teach and heal. We are told that they were filled with wonder *"when they saw the dumb, speak, and the maimed to be whole, the lame to walk, and the blind to see: and they glorified the God of Israel"* (Matthew 15:31).

You can imagine their excitement. Perhaps a brother, friend, or neighbor who was deaf was able to hear; a blind person was able to see!

In fact, they were so involved with what God was doing that three days went by! Sometimes we wonder when our pastor talks for three hours! I have a feeling that just about the time someone had started to think about food, God worked another mighty miracle. And everyone began glorifying God again and forgot about eating.

Our Lord's Real Concern

After three days, when Jesus finished healing and

43

teaching, He became concerned about the multitudes, *"Because they continue with me now three days, and have nothing to eat: and I will not send them away fasting, lest they faint in the way"* (Matthew 16:32). You can understand His concern since they still had a long walk back to the coasts of Tyre and Sidon. I love it that Jesus never forgets we live in a human body. He showed us often that He cares about our physical needs. Yet, He did not stop just because it was "time to eat."

Two Meals

As I began to eat only from *real hunger,* I soon found that I rarely wanted to eat lunch. I began to plan activities to use the time that I formerly spent planning and eating lunch. I ate breakfast, then dinner. I found that by eating only two meals a day, I could eat whatever I wanted for breakfast and dinner, yet the pounds came off.

Rather than count calories or carbohydrates, I ate whatever I desired. *But only if I was truly hungry.* I stopped eating when I felt full. I stopped using "diet" products. For the first time I began to eat more satisfying, regular foods. My focus began to change from, "What am I going to *eat* today?" to "What am I going to *do* today?" I began to seek God's purpose for each day and was thrilled to discover He had purpose and meaning for every day.

I began to lose that bloated feeling, "like I

44

needed to drink a bottle of Drano," as one woman so aptly put it. I found I had more energy and more time. I was much more productive and more mentally alert. *That awful, dragging, tiredness began to leave.*

Alert On An Empty Stomach

After eating this way for many years, it is interesting to read how many ministers and evangelists do not eat before they teach. They say they recall the Word better and are more alert mentally when their stomach is empty. There are times now, when we have out-of-town company, when I must go back into the three meals a day pattern. Frankly, I can't wait to get back to two meals a day.

I am astounded by the extent we have built our lives around food and eating! Our priorities need to be more like John the Baptist's who was happy eating locusts and wild honey. There was nothing sacred about eating locusts and wild honey; John ate to live—he didn't live to eat.

I also found that when eating from *real hunger* I tended to desire more healthful foods. A person who is having a real hunger response will not desire candy bars or cookies. They want meat, vegetables, milk, and bread.

I eat sweets when I want them; I have dessert when I want it; but I have found my desire for them has diminished. Chocolate doesn't even look good to me most of the time, but if I want some I eat some. *I just don't eat it to my condemnation anymore.* Praise God!

Really Enjoying Your Food

When a person begins to eat from hunger instead of the other reasons we mentioned, their appetite begins to change. I often prefer a cucumber more than anything else. But if I want a chocolate chip cookie, I don't hesitate to eat one. Food is not the culprit—overeating is. *No foods are restricted.* You see, God's plan is freedom. *I* control my eating, it doesn't control me anymore. I enjoy food much more than I ever did. When you have not eaten since breakfast, dinner looks delicious! I thank God for my food with a sincere heart. I really appreciate it.

It is a universal reaction in our classes that as people begin to eat only from *real hunger*, they experience a new enjoyment of their food. They marvel at the amount of food they were eating when they were not even hungry!

How Did God Feed?

I don't know exactly where today's "three-meal-a-day-clean-up-your-plate" eating philosophy originated, but it is *not* the pattern that God Himself used when He supernaturally fed men. When we look for spiritual examples of God supernaturally feeding His people, there is a consistent pattern.

In Exodus 16:12 God supernaturally provided

food for the Israelites. They were given two meals a day, *"At even ye shall eat flesh and in the morning ye shall be filled with bread."* In fact, their food was provided in such a way that it could only be eaten twice a day even if they wanted to eat three times a day.

We are told that after the morning meal, *"as the sun waxed hot, it melted"* (Exodus 16:21). In the evening they were specifically told to *"let no man leave of it til morning"* (Exodus 16:19). A few of the Israelites, probably the gluttons, decided to try to save a little. They found it had bred worms and began to stink. That would spoil your appetite for a bedtime snack!

How God Led Elijah And Aaron

In 1 Kings 17:4-6, we again see an example of God's supernatural feeding. This time He fed His mighty prophet Elijah. Again He gave food twice a day. *"And the ravens brought him bread and flesh in the morning and bread and flesh in the evening."* This time there was neither melting nor breeding of worms, but I am sure Elijah already had his priorities straight as far as eating was concerned. He was eating to live, not living to eat.

When God established the order of the sacrificial offerings in Exodus 29, although He did not supernaturally provide the food, He did set the rules. Again we see this consistent pattern of morning and evening meals. Aaron and his sons

47

were to take their food from certain parts of the sacrificial offering.

Bread was to be provided in a basket, by the door of the tabernacle of the congregation. *"And Aaron and his sons shall eat the flesh of the ram, and the bread that is in the basket, by the door of the tabernacle of the congregation"* (Exodus 29:32). *"The one lamb thou shalt offer in the morning: and the other lamb thou shalt offer at even"* (Exodus 29:39). When Jesus multiplied the loaves and fishes, he never stopped because it was "time to eat."

God's Practicality

There is nothing holy about eating two meals a day or sinful about eating three meals a day. I simply believe it is a very practical, good way to eat. I believe that God's way is always the best way.

It is readily apparent why this plan would allow a person to eat with more freedom. When you consider the number of calories per day a person may eat to maintain a certain weight, it makes sense. For example, I am 5'9", and weigh 137 pounds. I will be able to eat about 2000 calories a day for the rest of my life. This amount will drop slightly around the age of 55, but basically it will remain the same.

God is not going to change this basic amount of calories because there is nothing wrong with this amount. I am going to need this basic amount of calories for the rest of my natural life. If that 2000 calories is divided three ways, I can eat just over 660 calories per meal.

Typical Meal

For example, a breakfast of cereal with milk and a little sugar has 210 calories. Add orange juice and you add another 80-100 calories. For lunch, a chef's salad (the dieter's favorite) with dressing is about 1000 calories. Add a few crackers—another 50 calories. And because you were so good and ate a salad, you have dessert—another 250 calories, leaving about 400 calories left for the evening meal. That means you can eat a delicious meal of thin soup, dry toast, skim milk, and maybe an apple. That's not my idea of a lifetime eating pattern!

With that very same number of calories divided into two meals, there are plenty of calories for you to eat a solid breakfast with 1500 calories for dinner. This means that going out to dinner will not throw you off, having dessert with your meal will not throw you off, and eating ice cream with the kids will not throw you off. You have real freedom with your eating. Freedom to enjoy your food and do as Christ told His disciples. *"Eat such things as are set before you"* (Luke 10:8).

The most important advantage, of course, is that you are no longer counting calories or worrying about which foods are fattening. *You are able to keep your mind off of food. Food takes its proper place in your life again.* You begin to eat only when you are hungry and enjoy the food you eat.

Full Response

When I begin to talk about our equally important full response, people often ask me, "How much can I eat?" You can eat until you are filled. When God fed the Israelites, He said, *"Ye shall be filled with bread"* (Exodus 16:12). When Jesus multiplied the loaves and fishes, the people *"did all eat and were filled"*(Matthew 15:37).Again in John 6, *"And likewise of the fishes as much as they would. . . .When they were filled he said unto his disciples, Gather up the fragments that remain, that nothing be lost"* (John 6:11,12).

We should also note that in each case there were *leftovers;* seven basketfuls one time, and twelve basketfuls the next. Eat until you are full, *but no more.* Forget about cleaning up your plate. "Hungry" and "full" are your *God-given* responses. "Clean up your plate" is a *mom-given* response.

People often use the quote, "Waste not, want not" with regard to food left on a plate as though it was scriptural. The only problem is that this quote is not from Scripture—it is from Ben Franklin!

Your Individual Response

When Jesus fed the multitudes, in each case He *took up* the fragments that no food would be wasted. He did not have the people *eat* the fragments so that none would be wasted. In a restaurant, sometimes we are served more food than we can or should eat. Does that mean we should eat it? *No!* Eat until you are full, but no more.

You will be astonished when you realize how much food is eaten only because somebody else put it on our plates. God gave *you* your hungry and full responses, not the chef at the restaurant, not the friend who loaded your plate with food at a dinner party.

Dr. Gabe Mirkin, of the nationally syndicated radio station KMOX, put it this way, "When you eat beyond full, all you get is fat!"

Only What Is Sufficient

Sometimes I buy an ice cream cone, and even the smallest can be too much. Other times it is not. If it is too much for me, do I still eat it? No—I eat until I am filled, and no more.

Proverbs 25:16 tells us, *"Hast thou found honey? Eat so much as is sufficient for thee."* Again, God gave you your full response, not the ice cream or candy bar makers. Your full response will not remain the same all the time. Just as our caloric needs change, so our full response will change from day to day. Just eat "so much as is sufficient," and don't eat beyond your God-given full response.

Another popular theory used to justify eating beyond our full response is, "Think of the hungry children in India." Our prayers of intercession and

God's Word going forth will save the hungry children in India. *The fact that we do or do not clean our plates has absolutely zero effect on the hungry children in India!*

Filled Versus Stuffed

You will find that as you follow the two meal a day pattern on a consistent basis, your appetite will become smaller. You will gradually require less food, although you are still eating until you are filled. Filled does not mean *stuffed,* but filled does mean you have satisfied your stomach's hunger response.

In the beginning, eating until you are filled may still require quite a bit of eating. But stop eating when you are filled. The amount will lessen if you are faithful in your daily fasting. You are retraining your body to listen for your God-given hungry and full responses.

It is important to understand that these two responses, hungry and full, operate *in conjuction with one another,* not independent of one another. In other words, in order for your full response to function, you must be hungry when you begin eating. When a person begins to eat without being hungry, they begin to lose their sense of full.

Since there is no full response to shut off the desire for food, a person continues to eat without reaching a point where they no longer desire food. They continue eating until their stomach is literally stuffed. *This is not a full response.* A full response comes when your body has consumed enough calories to meet its needs.

Response And Desire For Food

When your full response is working properly, you will reach a point where you feel you can't eat another bite. You lose interest in the food and nothing set before you seems tempting. In fact, the thought of having to eat more food at this time should be somewhat sickening to you. Your response functions as God intended it to; it shuts off your desire for food in a very effective way.

In America, where food is so plentiful and servings very large, a full response usually comes before you have eaten everything on your plate. *If you are having seconds on a consistent basis, your full response is not in operation!* A full response probably comes before you have eaten everything on your plate. A stuffed response comes after you have eaten everything on the table!

The Bible calls this type of response "well filled" as opposed to simply being filled. In Psalm 78:29-31, we see that this type of eating is where gluttony begins. *"So they did eat, and were well filled: for he gave them their own desire; they were not estranged from their lust* (lusting for food). *But while their meat was yet in their mouths, the wrath of God came upon them, and slew the fattest of them. . ."*

Taking Up Your Fragments

If you have trouble continuing to eat even after you are really satisfied, take your plate and run water over it. Get the other food off the table as soon as possible. Don't just sit and nibble. Remember they *took up* the fragments that were left, they did not *eat up* the fragments. (See John 6.) Take away the food as an act of choosing God in your eating and offer it as seed.

The same principle can be used in a restaurant. If you continue to eat french fries, even when you know you have eaten enough, take your water glass and pour a little water on them. This will kill your appetite for them. The waitress may think you are a little strange, but what do you care if it helps you not to overeat!

Offer it to God. "Father, I choose not to overeat, and I pour this water over these french fries as a way of choosing You in my eating. I offer it to You as seed to the Spirit rather than the flesh."

Although we are born with these responses and do not have to learn them as children, when we have lost them as adults, *we must relearn them*. We must learn what it feels like to have our stomach empty—to experience real hunger. Often after years of dieting, we feel that it is always all right to eat some types of food such as celery or carrot sticks.

This type of eating, while not high in calories, does not allow you to recognize your hungry and full responses. It does not deal with the gluttony. A person is still turning to food, but it is low calorie food instead of high calorie food. It may lead to some control, but never *freedom*.

Real Hunger Is Easily Satisfied

Most people are amazed at how little food they actually need to eat after having overeaten for many years. One man came late to class and only heard the last thirty minutes of this teaching on hungry and full. He went home, however, and applied what he heard. By the next week he had lost ten pounds by doing nothing but eating only when he was hungry!

People are often astounded in class to learn they have lost weight. I remember one woman who gave excuses all the way to the scales. She said that all she did was not eat when she wasn't hungry, and she probably hadn't lost any weight. Her face certainly came alive when she saw she had lost three pounds that week and didn't even know it!

When a person has struggled so much with their weight, drawing on all their will power and constraining themselves to the very limit of their endurance to take off weight, they are utterly unprepared for the "easy yoke" when Jesus is in it with them. I frequently receive calls expressing concern because it is too easy. They actually want to know what is wrong!

Drastic Drop In Appetite

People also become concerned when they have a drastic decrease in appetite. This excerpt from a letter I recently received is not an infrequent response. "I felt I wasn't getting enough to eat! I could only eat half of a banana and half of a sandwich, and that was a challenge." Another lady, who had over sixty pounds to lose, said she was worried because she could only eat about half of what was on her plate.

A person who is sixty pounds overweight has 210,000—or *almost a quarter of a million stored calories* (in the form of fat). *Expect a drastic decrease in your appetite* as you begin to eat from your God-given hungry and full responses. Count on it—watch for it—rejoice in it!

The following chart will help you understand why your appetite will decrease significantly. It also helps illustrate why too much weight is a strain on the body and why it saps vital energy.

STORED CALORIES PER POUND OF OVERWEIGHT
by Diane Hampton

Pounds of Overweight	Stored Calories Of Fat	Days Of Stored Calories	Months Of Stored Calories
5	17,500	8.75	
10	35,000	17.5	
15	52,500	26.25	

20	70,000	35.00	1.1
25	87,500	43.75	1.45
30	105,000	52.5	1.72
35	122,500	61.25	2.00
40	140,000	70.00	2.30
45	157,500	78.75	2.58
50	175,000	87.50	2.87
55	192,500	96.25	3.15
60	210,000	105.00	3.44
65	227,500	113.75	3.73
70	245,000	122.50	4.02
75	262,500	131.25	4.30
80	280,000	140.00	4.59
85	297,500	148.75	4.88
90	315,000	157.50	5.16
95	332,500	166.25	5.45
100	350,000	175.00	5.73
105	367,500	183.75	6.02
110	385,000	192.50	6.31

Based on caloric needs of approximately 2000 calories a day and 3500 calories per one pound of excess weight.

While our bodies store fat, *they cannot store many needed vitamins.* Just because you have a month's stored fat does not mean you have a month's stored vitamins and minerals. However, this chart helps us understand the decrease in appetite and feel more comfortable with it.

The "Easy Yoke"

Last year we went on a cruise. Anyone who has been on a cruise knows the lavish meals they serve. Every meal was a feast! Toward the end of the cruise, some of the passengers were waddling on the decks, stuffed to the gills, yet dreading the inevitable diets they anticipated on their return home. I ate anything I wanted throughout the entire cruise and thoroughly enjoyed the food, but I didn't gain a pound.

Before I went in for a meal, I considered, "Am I really hungry?" If the answer was, "No," I did not even go into the dining room. This was almost always the noon meal. Don and I would walk the decks, shop, or do something else.

When evening came, we were ready to eat! I'll bet our food tasted better than anyone else's because we allowed ourselves to become hungry before we ate. It is not unusual for people to come back from vacations taken during the classes with the report that they lost weight. They lost this weight even though they ate every meal at a restaurant!

One woman beamed to discover she lost three pounds over her vacation. And she never ate any special foods or diet menus. *Freedom.* Another woman, over forty years of age, reported that for the first time in her life, she did not gain weight over the Thanksgiving holiday. Yet, she ate everything to her satisfaction.

Compensating For A Large Meal

Eating only when you are hungry, after having eaten a large meal the previous evening, can mean not eating until the evening meal the next day. You will not become hungry until your body needs fuel again, and that will be longer than normal when you have eaten more. In other words, if you have eaten more than your daily caloric needs in one meal, don't eat with your usual pattern the next day. Allow your body to use up the extra calories by waiting until you are hungry.

Some Common Changes

God created our bodies perfectly. He created them to live in health and fellowship with Him. After one of our classes, we asked the men and women to write down some of the changes that had come about in their lives as they brought their eating into line with the Word of God.

Over and over they mentioned they had more fellowship with God. They found that they easily adjusted to fewer meals, they were more active, more productive, had a new enjoyment for life, were more obedient in other areas, watched less TV, and found it much easier to fast when they were called to fast for other reasons.

They also mentioned how their faith had grown to believe God for other things as they see victory in their weight. The direction and focus of their lives changed from food to fellowship, and it is a wonderful change!

Chapter 5

RESISTING TEMPTATION

Scripture tells us, *"Submit yourselves therefore to God"* (James 4:7). When you offer this daily fasting to God, you are submitting yourself and your eating to God. Tell God you are submitting your eating to Him this day. "Father I choose You in my eating today. I choose Your will for my life. I will sow seed to the Spirit this day and not to the flesh."

The second part of this Scripture says, *"Resist the devil and he will flee from you."* To resist means to "strive against or oppose, to make a stand or effort in opposition." It does not mean to stand in a nose-to-nose confrontation. If you sit and think about a piece of blueberry pie to see how long you can hold out, you're not going to make it very long.

Eating And Non-Eating Activities

God showed me that there were certain times and activities when I consistently tended to overeat. Conversely, there were certain times and activities when I consistently tended to forget about eating.

Take a sheet of paper and make a list called, "Activities When I Consistently Tend to Overeat." For example many people tend to overeat while watching TV at night or during the afternoon. Perhaps a problem time is when you are bored or overtired.

On another sheet of paper make a list called, "Activities When I Consistently Tend To Forget About Eating." For example, cleaning out a closet, working in the yard, or listening to Christian tapes. Spend some time and thought in making this list—don't try to do it all in ten minutes.

One way of sowing to the Spirit and resisting the devil is to consciously choose to move from an "eating activity" to a "non-eating activity." If you have trouble eating when you are in your house alone, one way of sowing to the Spirit is to choose to get out of your house (go visit a friend in the hospital, take a walk around the block) and offer it to God as seed. "Father, You know that I would like to eat right now, but I choose to get out of the house instead, and I offer this to You as seed."

If you have trouble eating when you watch TV at night, choose to do handwork or take a bath instead.

Choosing To Sow Seed

There is nothing holy about taking a walk or

doing handwork. It is when you purposely choose to do these activities instead of eating and offer it to God as a way of choosing Him in your eating that you have sown seed to the Spirit. Proverbs 16:2 tells us, "All the ways of a man are clean in his own eyes; but the Lord weigheth the spirits." Avoid activities which usually lead to overeating, even if they seem right with your natural eye. God weighs the spirits, He knows that you know the activity leads to overeating.

Get your focus off what you are eating or not eating. Focus on which activities lead to eating and which activities do not. As God begins to reveal this to you, use your power of choice wisely. The Bible clearly teaches that the choices we make affect our freedom.

"Enter not into the path of the wicked (a situation that usually leads to overeating). . .*Avoid it, pass not by it, turn from it, and pass away"* Proverbs 4:14,15).

"(You) *Ponder the path of thy feet, and let all thy ways be established"* (Proverbs 4:26). Establish in this verse means to "cause to be or happen; bring about." Plan your daily activities around *not eating.*

"The highway of the upright is to depart from evil: he that keepeth his way preserveth his soul" (Proverbs 16:17).

Understanding And Wisdom From God

One of the ways I was able to control overeating

was to stop staying up late at night. I liked to watch the late movie. In fact, I learned that any time I stayed up late, I was much more likely to overeat the next day. Once I understood this, I began to "ponder the path of (my) feet" and establish my way. I did this by going to bed earlier instead of watching the late movie. Now there is nothing wrong with staying up late at night, but the *"Lord weigheth the spirits,"* and for me, keeping late hours led to overeating.

With my healing, I received wisdom from God with regard to my eating. My healing has continued over eleven years because God gave me wisdom. *"Out of his mouth cometh knowledge and understanding* (with regard to eating). *He layeth up sound wisdom for the righteous: he is a buckler to them that walk uprightly. He keepeth the paths of judgment, and preserveth the way of his saints. Then shalt thou understand righteousness...* (He not only healed me, He showed me how He intended me to eat, what type of eating leads to gluttony, and what type does not.) *When wisdom entereth into thine heart, and knowledge is pleasant unto thy soul; discretion shall preserve thee, understanding shall keep thee"* (Proverbs 2:6-10).

What Is Discretion?

Discretion means the freedom or authority to make decisions and choices. God's Word says that this discretion shall preserve you. When you are trapped in gluttony or compulsive eating—or any compulsive behavior—your choices are hidden from you. God returns your freedom of choice, but He leaves the final choice with you. Your discretion will keep, or preserve, you in freedom. I know that I will never have a problem with eating again for the rest of my life because I make choices every day according to the wisdom God gave me regarding food. How much better to have understanding and weight loss rather than just weight loss.

Keeping Your House Clean

Jesus warned us, *"When the unclean spirit is gone out of a man* (as the spirit of overeating), *he walketh through dry places, seeking rest, and findeth none. Then he saith, I will return into my house from whence I came out* (you); *and when he is come he findeth it empty* (still sitting there watching TV thinking about food), *swept and garnished* (ripe for a binge). *Then goeth he, and taketh with him seven other spirits more wicked than himself* (Mr. Binge, Mr. Condemnation, Mr. Depression, etc.) *and they enter in and dwell there; and the last state of that man is worse than the first"* (Matthew 12:43-45).

Don't let Satan come back to find your house empty! Let him find you full of the Word and moving out in faith to another activity. Resist the devil. If you resist, he must flee from you.

Changing from eating to non-eating activities is

65

not just a good thing to do, *it is a vital part of your healing*. Jesus warns us in this parable that if we leave our house empty, if we don't fill that part of our life with something meaningful, then we are open prey for the same wicked spirits to return, stronger than before.

How To Change Your Ways

If you have trouble because you eat after dinner, night after night, *Repent!* Repent means to *"think differently."* Change the way you think about your time after dinner. Start taking walks, play a family game, or start a hobby that keeps your hands busy. Replace the old, negative pattern in your life with something positive. Plan other activities during the time you used to have a problem with eating.

For example, I always try to schedule all appointments around the noon hour. This is an old habit I picked up during the time of my healing (sow an action, reap a habit). I learned that if I had an activity planned for the time I had trouble with eating, I would fast much more easily. I learned to "keep my way" in order to preserve my soul.

Choosing The Right Activity

Make your activity something you can look forward to. As much as possible, make it involve other people. Be creative in your ideas. I found that planning more activities outside in the fresh air helped.

Sometimes we must fill our empty house with the Word of God. David said of God, *"Thou art my hiding place, thou shalt preserve me from trouble; thou shalt compass me about with songs of deliverance. . . . What time I am afraid, I will trust in thee"* (Psalms 32:7, 56:3). God's Word is our "song of deliverance." Our souls can hide in it when we are afraid.

When I was worried, instead of turning to food as I had before, I read, *"Trust in the Lord with all thine heart; and lean not unto thine own understanding"* (Proverbs 3:5). God's Word ministered to my spirit, and I was able to stop worrying. When I felt depression coming, instead of eating I read, *"For God hath not given us the spirit of fear; but of power, and of love, and of a sound mind"* (2 Timothy 1:7).

Instead of fighting with a knife and fork, I began to do battle with the sword of the Word. It ministered to my spirit, and I was able to resist depression.

When I was angry at others or myself, instead of eating I would read, *"Renew a right spirit within me"* (Psalm 51:10), and *"if ye forgive not men their trespasses, neither will your Father forgive your trespasses"* (Matthew 6:15). I always said in my heart, *"God knows why I am angry. He knows what they did to me. I don't get mad without a good reason."* When I saw from God's Word that it didn't mention whether or not I had a good reason, I became serious about forgiving.

67

I found that as I began to forgive others, I was able to forgive myself. God's Word is health, purity, truth, and righteousness.

A Just Man Falleth Seven Times

What if you begin the day, commit your eating to God, and all goes well until about 10:00 a.m.? Then you begin to eat. My healing was not overnight. It took a period of months, and sometimes I fell back into compulsive eating during those months.

First of all, you can expect Satan to be there with condemnation if you do start to overeat again. He will tell you, "You have blown it. You might as well go ahead and eat." He will tell you what a failure you are, and that this isn't going to work any better than any other diet.

But God's Word says, *"the just man falleth seven times, and riseth up again"* (Proverbs 24:16). Being perfect before God is not a matter of never falling—*it is a question of what you do about it when you do fall.* A just man rises up again!

Why do you think condemnation is such a favorite tool of the devil? Because he knows if he can get you into condemnation rather than repentance, he can probably keep you from going to God. Satan likes nothing better than to tell us we have really blown it, and we had better not go before God after what we've done.

When we have overeaten (or done anything else

sinful), we feel the least like going before God. We don't even want to be around other people. But this is the most important time to go to God.

Is It Too Late For A New Beginning?

You have not blown it. You are not on a diet so you can't blow it! Tell yourself, "I have sown to the flesh but I will not say that I have blown it and continue to sow to the flesh. I repent, Father, and I resolve right now, *this hour,* to sow to the Spirit. I thank You, Father, that it is never too late for a new beginning. This day may have started in defeat, but it will end in victory!

Remember the woman who was caught in the act of adultery? The people wanted to stone her, but when she was brought before Jesus, He said, *"Neither do I condemn thee: go, and sin no more"* (John 8:11). If you will go to God right in the middle of a binge and repent, His answer will be the same. *"Neither do I condemn you,"* and you will be able to *"go, and sin no more."*

You see, when that woman repented, she chose Jesus, and power was released into her life to go and sin no more. That same power will be released into your life. You have God's Word on it. He promised, *"But as many as received him to them gave he power to become the sons of God"* (John 1:12). Purpose in your heart to commit your eating to God and redirect the focus of your life away from food.

Re-Creating Eating Patterns

On the following pages are what we call "Seven Days of Re-Creating Your Eating Patterns." Each day there is a prayer to commit that day's eating to God. There is a space to write down what you resolve to do that day instead of eating. It is important for your success that you decide each day what you are going to do as seed to the Spirit.

You have spent much time and planning on what you were going to *eat* for the last few years. Now spend some time planning what you are going to *do*. Remember that God has a purpose and plan for each life, and it never includes overeating.

These activities can be things such as going to visit someone in the hospital, cleaning out a closet, meeting a new neighbor, or doing handwork. Proverbs 31:13 tells us that a virtuous woman *"worketh willingly with her hands."* These are all seeds to the Spirit, because you are purposing in your heart, before God, to do these activities *instead of eating*.

There is also a commitment to read confessions each day about your eating, and a commitment to thank God for everything you ate that day. (There will be more about these last two commitments in subsequent chapters.)

Don't leave these spaces blank. Decide what seeds you are going to sow each day, write them in, then do them. If you begin to fall back into poor eating habits, don't let Satan tell you where you have failed for the day. Start from that hour as though it were a new day.

One of the greatest joys I had during my time of healing was when I began a binge, realized what I was doing, and then made a decision to choose God. I never finished the binge. That was when I knew I was being healed.

DAY 1

Father, I commit my eating to You today. Beginning this day, I will seek a new eating pattern for me that will last for the rest of my life. I seek a change in my whole attitude about food and my appetite. Your Word says, *"he that soweth to the Spirit shall of the Spirit reap"* (Galatians 6:8), and so I offer You my seed to eat only two meals this day. You promised power to as many as received You. I receive You this day in my eating, and I receive power to walk as a son of God in my eating. Seed to the Spirit:

Instead of eating lunch or dinner (circle one) this day I will _____

_____

_____

and I offer this to You, Lord, as seed to the Spirit.

Instead of bedtime eating this day I will _____

_____

72

and I offer this to You, Lord, as seed to the Spirit.

I will offer thanksgiving to You for everything I eat today because Your Word says that my food is sanctified by this thanksgiving.

I will read my confessions from Your Word this day and my confessions about my weight.

DAY 2

Father, I commit my eating to You today. Fill this day with Your purpose and meaning. I will sow seed to the Spirit today to set a new eating pattern in my life. I receive You this day in my eating, and I receive power to walk as a son of God. Father, I thank You that Your Word is supernatural. Because it is supernatural, I will have supernatural help when I choose You in my eating. Seed to the Spirit:

Instead of eating lunch or dinner (circle one) this day I will _____

_____

_____

and I offer this to You, Lord, as seed to the Spirit.

Instead of bedtime eating this day I will _____

_____

_____

and I offer this to You, Lord, as seed to the Spirit.

I will offer thanksgiving to You for everything I

eat today because Your Word says my food is sanctified by this thanksgiving.

I will read positive confessions about my eating today, and I will meditate on Your Word when I am lonely, worried, frustrated, angry, or experiencing other negative emotions.

DAY 3

Father, I commit my eating to You today. Beginning this day, I will seek a new eating pattern for me that will last for the rest of my life. I will seek a change in my whole attitude about food and my appetite. Your Word says that he who *"soweth to the Spirit shall of the Spirit reap."* So I offer You my seed to eat only two meals this day. You promised power to as many as received You. I receive You this day in my eating, and I receive power to walk as a son of God in my eating. Seed to the Spirit:

Instead of eating lunch or dinner (circle one) this day I will _____

_____

_____

and I offer this to You, Lord, as seed to the Spirit.

Instead of bedtime eating this day I will _____

_____

76

and I offer this to You, Lord, as seed to the Spirit.

I will offer thanksgiving to You for everything I eat today because Your Word says my food is sanctified by this thanksgiving.

I will read my confessions from Your Word this day and my confessions about my weight.

DAY 4

Father, I commit my eating to You today. Fill this day with Your purpose and meaning. I will sow seed to the Spirit today to set a new eating pattern in my life. I receive You this day in my eating, and I receive power to walk as a son of God in my eating. Father, I thank You that Your Word is supernatural, and so I will have supernatural help when I choose You in my eating. Seed to the Spirit:

Instead of eating lunch or dinner (circle one) this day I will _____

_____

_____

and I offer this to You, Lord, as seed to the Spirit.

Instead of bedtime eating this day I will _____

_____

_____

and I offer this to You, Lord, as seed to the Spirit.

I will offer thanksgiving to You for everything I

eat today because Your Word says my food is sanctified by this thanksgiving.

I will read my confessions about my eating today, and I will meditate on Your Word when I am lonely, frustrated, worried, angry, or experiencing any other negative emotion.

DAY 5

Father, I commit my eating to You today. I choose obedience. Jesus said, *"if ye love me, keep my commandments"* (John 14:15), and I love You, Lord, so I will not eat to my condemnation. I will sow seed to the Spirit that I may reap of the Spirit. Seed to the Spirit:

Instead of eating lunch or dinner (circle one) this day I will _____

_____

_____

and I offer it to You, Lord, as seed to the Spirit.

Instead of bedtime eating this day I will _____

_____

_____

and I offer this to You, Lord, as seed to the Spirit.

I will offer thanksgiving to You for everything I eat today because Your Word says my food is sanctified by this thanksgiving.

I will read positive confessions about my eating

today, and I will meditate on Your Word when I am lonely, worried, frustrated, or angry.

DAY 6

Father, I commit my eating to You today. You know that this is a weekend, Father, and so I ask for special help today. I ask You for special purpose for this day. I will sow seed to the Spirit today and expect to reap from the Spirit. I receive You in my eating today, and I thank You for power to walk as a son of God in my eating this day. Seed to the Spirit:

Instead of eating lunch or dinner (circle one) I will _____

_____

_____

and I offer this to You, Lord, as seed to the Spirit.

Instead of bedtime eating this day I will _____

_____

_____

and I offer this to You, Lord, as seed to the Spirit.

I will offer thanksgiving to You for everything I

eat today because Your Word says my food is sanctified by this thanksgiving.

I will read my confessions about my eating today from Your Word.

DAY 7

Father, I commit my eating to You today. I thank You for a sabbath day of rest. I thank You that gluttony is losing its power in my life because I am choosing You in my eating. I thank You for the power and freedom to walk as a son of God this day.

I will offer You thanksgiving for everything I eat this day because Your Word says my food is sanctified by this thanksgiving.

I will read my confessions today.

What To Expect From Your Seed

When you plant a seed in the ground, it will not come up the next day. In fact, you will not see anything happen for a week to ten days. You have to watch and believe the seed is growing. After a week or ten days, you begin to see a tiny sprout pushing up out of the ground.

It will be the same with your fasting. There will be a time at the beginning when it will seem like nothing is happening. That is the time we must stand in faith. Do not stop making your daily commitment to God. God's Word says something will happen, *and it will happen.*

After a period you will begin to see the "sprout" in your life, you will notice food is losing its control over you. Chocolate will stop looking so good. Things which were so hard to pass up will become easier and easier to not eat. You will begin to be free indeed.

When To Set Fasting Goals

If at any point, the fasting becomes too heavy, go back to the hungry and full pattern. If you find yourself setting fasting goals you are not meeting, go back to asking yourself before you eat anything, "Am I really hungry?" Don't set a fasting goal for yourself at this time.

When Jesus is in the yoke with you, fasting will not be a difficult thing. Remember, Jesus said if we are faithful in that which is least, we will be faithful in much. Go back to where you can be faithful and be sensitive to the change in your appetite when it comes. You will begin to experience a supernatural ability to fast. That is the time to get back to fasting.

Chapter 6

TRANSFORMED BY NEW THOUGHTS

Most Christians have heard Mark 11:23,24 quoted many times. *"Whosoever shall say unto this mountain, Be thou removed, and be thou cast into the sea; and shall not doubt in his heart, but shall believe that those things which he saith shall come to pass; he shall have whatsoever he saith."* It is one of the great truths of God.

But did you know this same truth can work in a negative way? Remember when Jesus walked by the fig tree without fruit, and He cursed it saying, *"No man eat fruit of thee hereafter for ever"* (Mark 11:14)? I used to wonder why Jesus would curse a poor, old fig tree. He was teaching us that faith can work in a negative way also. The next day when the disciples passed the fig tree, they marveled because it was dried up from the roots, but Jesus said, *"He shall have whatsoever he saith."*

Cursing Your Fig Tree

Some people have been cursing their fig trees

with regard to their weight for many years. "I just can't seem to lose weight. I came from an overweight family. I guess I will always be fat. I can look at food and gain weight." Yet, Proverbs 13:2 says, *"A man shall eat good by the fruit of his mouth."* Proverbs 18:20 says, *"A man's belly shall be satisfied with the fruit of his mouth."*

Paul's admonition in Romans 12:2 to *"be not conformed to this world: but be ye transformed by the renewing of your mind"* coincides with the truth that our words are creative. If we renew our minds and uplift our thoughts, our words will also be uplifting.

Some words build us up inside. When I am discouraged, or something seems overwhelming to me, I say, *"I can do all things through Christ which strengtheneth me"* (Phillipians 4:13). That Scripture reaches down inside me and lifts me up. My posture gets a little straighter, and I know I am going to make it. I have done things I would have sworn were impossible by stepping out in faith on this Scripture.

Some words fill up your soul. Proverbs 27:7 tells us, *"A full soul loatheth a honeycomb."* If your soul is full, even a honeycomb (today it might be a Hershey chocolate bar) isn't tempting. This proverb also warns, *"to the hungry soul, every bitter thing is sweet."*

If your soul is hungry, if you feel turmoil inside, you will want to eat everything. Even unappetizing things will seem sweet. When you feel discouragement emptying your soul, have some food for the soul ready.

Word To Fill Your Soul

Saying, "I can't seem to lose weight" empties your soul. Saying, "Those things which are impossible with men are possible with God" fills your soul. Instead of saying, "I can't seem to lose weight" say, "I lose weight easily." Instead of saying, "I have been overweight all my life" say, "I am thin." Here are some more positive faith statements about weight which you might use:

"I can do all things through Christ which strengtheneth me" (Philippians 4:13). I can lose weight and control my eating for the rest of my life through Christ.

My appetite is being totally changed through Jesus my Lord. Jesus, *"who his own self bore our sins in his own body. . .that I might be dead to sins"* (gluttony) (1 Peter 2:24).

I receive Jesus in my eating, so I receive *"Power to (become the sons) of God"* (John 1:12).

I wear a size _____ (goal size).

I weigh _____ (goal weight).

You may use any of these confessions or make up a list of your own. Begin to repeat healing Scriptures aloud each day. Apply them to your weight. Remember, *"He shall have whatsoever he saith"* (Mark 11:23).

Old Things Are Passed Away

The devil is called the deceiver. He often tries to lead us into spiritual quicksand where we can get stuck. If we don't know the Word of God, we will begin to sink. There is a teaching today, a half-truth which is Satan's specialty. We read and hear about it every day of our lives. We are bombarded with this philosophy in the media, magazines, and newspapers. I think we need to evaluate it in light of God's Word.

The idea is that what we are today is completely determined by what happened to us in our childhood. In other words, *our past controls our future.* I see many examples of this type thinking in compulsive eaters.

A woman came to me for counseling one day. Her hair was dirty and unkept. She could hardly speak without breaking down in tears. Her eyes mirrored the hopelessness she felt. She had been to many counseling sessions with many counselors. She began the session by talking about her parents and her past, as I am sure she had so many times before.

I stopped her midway, and asked her if she was born again. She said she was. I responded, "Mary, I want to share some things with you from the Word of God. This may be very different from what you have heard before, but it has been very important in my own life, and I believe it will help you also."

I read to her from 2 Corinthians 5:17, *"If any man be in Christ, he is a new creature. Old things are passed away; behold, all things are become new."* I also shared Philippians 3:13,14 with her. *"But this one thing I do, forgetting those things which are behind, and reaching forth unto those things which are before, I press toward the mark for the prize of the high calling of God in Christ Jesus."* I explained to her that when she was born again, she became a new creature inside and that nothing from the past could control her future anymore.

I encouraged her to stop looking to the past for reasons for her problems, but rather to *"Put on the new man, which after God is created in righteousness"* (Ephesians 4:24). Rather than to continually drag out the past, we are told as new creatures to *"Put off concerning the former conversation the old man"* (Ephesians 4:22). In other words, quit dragging and start pressing! That is what the good news is all about. What a thrill to witness a life totally transformed by the power of Jesus Christ.

Joyful Results

She seemed surprised. She had been looking backward so long that she completely lost any vision for the future. Proverbs 29:18 says, *"Where there is no vision, the people perish."* She was perishing on the inside. I told her to wash her hair, use make-up on her face, and do a number of other things during the next week. I shared with her the principles of sowing to the Spirit and showed her how this applied to her particular problem.

The next week when she came back, even I was surprised. I didn't have to ask her how she had been that week. She glowed. The entire expression of her face had changed. She met me with a smile and her eyes were bright. What a change as she began to *"forget those things which are behind, and reach for those things which are before."*

One overweight Christian told me that she was overweight today because someone put a curse on her grandmother. Another shared that she was overweight because of her mother. Her mother was unhappy at the prospect of having a baby, a baby who turned out to be this woman. They were allowing their past to determine their future!

Stop looking for reasons for your compulsive eating. God never directed me backward—*only forward.* There was no hidden, secret reason behind my eating. I could not tell you today what caused my gluttony. But I can tell you today that I am free through Christ Jesus, and I'll take that anytime!

Trials Will Come

Another easy trap to fall into is to "wait until everything settles down" emotionally before you try to sow to the Spirit. I can assure you now that the devil will make sure things *never* settle down if that is all it takes to keep you from victory.

Jesus tells us, *"It is impossible but that offenses will come"* (Luke 17:1). He might have added, "And often!" As one need is met, another need arises. The steadying force is knowing, *"My God shall supply all your need according to his riches in glory by Christ Jesus"* (Philippians 4:19). The peace of God that surpasses understanding is knowing that God will meet your need as you look to Him.

You are going to have situations arise in your life that cause emotional upset. Jesus said that in the world we would have tribulation. You can count on it. You can plan on it! But He also said, *"Be of good cheer: I have overcome the world!"* (John 16:33).

My Story

In my own life, a couple of years after my healing, a situation arose which could have been disastrous to my healing. I was pregnant with our much wanted second child when I began to bleed. The doctors told me I only had a 50/50 chance of carrying the baby full term. Four or five times I was put on virtual bed rest for ten days at a time. This was nothing more than a subtle scheme of the devil to try to get me back into gluttony.

He laid the trap well. This was the closest I ever came to returning to compulsive eating. But as the Word says, *"Discretion shall preserve thee"*

(Proverbs 2:10). God, through His healing, returned discretion to me—the freedom or authority to make decisions—and this discretion preserved me.

This was a time when I could have been very bored, and it was a time of emotional pressure. Both are dangerous times for former gluttons. It was a time to, *"Put on the whole armour of God, that* (I) *may be able to stand against the wiles of the devil"* (Ephesians 6:11). I made a choice right then to *"Ponder the path of* (my) *feet, and let all* (my) *ways be established"* (Proverbs 4:26.) My armor went up!

Handling The Difficulty

I planned activities for this time, *from the first day,* that led me away from eating. I determined from the first day to sow several hours of fasting each day. I made sure I would not be alone most of the time. I invited friends to visit. As always, I read my Bible and spent time in prayer each day.

I made it through with flying colors! I didn't eat, I didn't lose the baby, and I knew from that moment forward that nothing would ever make me turn to food again—and it hasn't. That child is almost nine years old, but I have never been tempted to turn to food, to the praise and glory of God.

Don't let anything keep you from pressing toward the mark—especially the ups and downs of daily life.

Ecclesiastes 11:4 says, *"He that observeth the wind shall not sow; and he that regardeth the clouds shall not reap."* It goes on in verse 6 to say, *"In the morning sow thy seed."* If you are always observing your life, waiting until everything is normal to begin sowing, you will never reap. We want to wait for things to settle down and then confront our eating.

God's way is to confront our eating, knowing that afterwards things will settle down. We are told in Hebrews 12:1 to *"Let us lay aside every weight, and the sin which doth so easily beset us."* Which sin? The particular sin which attacks us so easily. For a glutton or a compulsive eater, the sin is using food the wrong way. Don't try to put this problem on a back burner.

Don't Be Overwhelmed

Perhaps laying aside this sin seems absolutely overwhelming to you. If you are feeling powerless to overcome it, you are looking at *your* ability and your past failures rather than to *God's* ability.

I received a letter recently from a person who was feeling overwhelmed by her problem with eating. She made a very frank and almost shocking statement. She said, "At times this obsession even supercedes God in my life." I know she was really feeling this, but I don't believe it was really true.

I believe she just felt overwhelmed by the power that food seemed to hold over her. I believe she was trying to take on the whole problem at once, and she didn't see how in the world she could make it. I shared with her a most important principle that Jesus taught us about the Kingdom of God. It is this, *"He that is faithful in that which is least is faithful also in much"* (Luke 16:10). Jesus is telling us to break down that problem to the point where we can be faithful.

God Supercedes Everything

This woman desperately needed to know that God *did* supercede her desire for food. She needed to grow to where she could be faithful. I told her to begin tomorrow doing the following— *and nothing else*—with regard to her eating.

Take the first ten things you are tempted to eat tomorrow (other than breakfast). Hold each one in your hand when you are being tempted. Hold just that one item up and ask yourself, "Who do you love more? This Oreo cookie or Jesus?" Do the same with the next thing you are tempted to eat until you have confronted ten foods.

I know what her response will be because I have used this so often in my own life. You see, she did love the Lord more, but the devil wants us to stay overwhelmed. God wants us to start where we can, but we must start.

Sometimes we try to move a giant tree when God only expects us to plant a seed. *You do what you can, and God will do what you cannot.*

Chapter 7

EAT WHATEVER IS SET BEFORE YOU

When a person has been on many diets for many years, he is likely to make food choices with calories or carbohydrates in mind. He is always buying special foods.

Some foods have come to be viewed as "good foods." If he is eating these foods, he feels he has eaten well. Other foods have come to be viewed as "bad foods." If he eats these foods, he feels condemnation. Too much of the wrong kind of importance is given to the foods he eats.

What about *what* we eat? What did Jesus teach about what we eat? Food fads, or so called "truths," come and go, but God's Word is truth itself. There are no higher findings than what Jesus Christ taught. His life is our example in every area. It reveals truth that we can count on, truth that will last.

What Did Jesus Teach About Eating?

People today are uptight about food. There is

97

hardly a food that isn't suspect in some circles. Bookshelves are filled with answers about what we should and shouldn't be eating. One eats sugar; another adamantly opposes it. One eats meat; another eats only vegetables. Relationships, even among family members and brothers in the Lord, can feel the strain of the diversity of beliefs.

I believe Jesus was very aware of the divisions such doctrines can cause. When He sent out the seventy disciples, He gave specific instructions with regard to *what* to eat. This would have been an ideal time to give instructions and laws regarding food.

Yet, His statements were simple and clear. *"In the same house remain, eating and drinking such things as they give. . .Eat such things as are set before you"* (Luke 10:7,8). In other words, whatever they are eating, you eat. Eat whatever is set before you.

In Matthew 15:11, Jesus said, *"Not that which goeth into the mouth defileth a man; but that which cometh out of the mouth, this defileth a man."* What goes into the mouth? Food! Man is not defiled by what he eats.

In fact, in Matthew 6:25, Jesus tells us to, *"Take no thought for your life, what ye shall eat, or what ye shall drink."* This is in strong contrast to a great deal of teaching which is going forth today, even in the Church. Today we hear, "take great thought about what you are to eat."

The Spirit Speaking Through Paul

Paul addresses the same subject with great consistency throughout his letters. In Colossians 2:16, he instructs us to *"Let no man therefore judge you in meat, or in drink."* He goes on to say, *"Wherefore if ye be dead with Christ from the rudiments of the world, why, as though living in the world, are ye subject to ordinances, touch not; taste not"* (Colossians 2:20). Paul was unmoved by doctrines coming forth that we shouldn't eat certain foods.

Spiritually, Paul tells us, *"But meat* (food) *commendeth us not to God: for neither, if we eat, are we the better; neither, if we eat not, are we the worse"* (1 Corinthians 8:8). *"For the kingdom of God is not meat and drink"* (Romans 14:17).

What About Nutrition And Health?

What about processed and nonprocessed foods? Some have taught that the reason Jesus was never sick was because He never ate processed foods.

Part of that is very true. Jesus did not eat processed food. *There were no processed foods at the time of Christ*—yet, *sickness was rampant!* If not eating processed foods was the secret of good health, there should have been no sickness in Jesus' time.

Even today, in countries where there are no processed foods, the life expectancy is only one-half of that in the United States. Nations without processed foods often face starvation and every form of sickness and disease, rather than experiencing the healthy life one would expect to find.

Importance Of Processed Foods

Of course, foods can be overprocessed. Sometimes nutritional value is needlessly lost, but other times nutritional value is greatly enhanced. Save an apple for three months (in its natural state) and examine the nutritional value of the rotted fruit. Take the same apple off the tree and process it quickly into apple sauce or frozen slices. Process it, save it for three months, and the comparative nutritional value of the apple is greatly enhanced by the processing. Ask our forefathers about the health benefits of trying to make it through the long winter months without processed foods.

Of all the sick people Jesus ministered to—and there were multitudes—*He never mentioned what they were eating.*

If what we eat is so important to our health, wouldn't Jesus have mentioned it to all the sick people He dealt with? He never indicated in any way that they needed to change what they were eating.

He did mention faith. *"Thy faith hath made thee whole. . . . According to your faith be it unto you. . . . Verily I say unto you, I have not found so great faith, no, not in Israel"* (Matthew 9:22,

9:29, and 8:10). He did not say, "I have not found so great a diet, no not in Israel."

Jesus ate as He instructed His disciples. He ate, "whatever (was) set before Him." When walking through a cornfield—when He was hungry—we are told that He plucked corn to eat. When He passed by a fig tree—and was hungry—He reached for a fig. When He multiplied the fish and loaves, He never changed what He multiplied. He multiplied whatever was set before Him.

Some believe they should eat Ezekiel's bread, but Jesus didn't. Some say we should eat as Daniel, only eating pulse (vegetables) and water. The Bible does say in Daniel 1:15, that Daniel and the children of Israel who did not eat the king's meat were *"fairer and fatter in flesh than all the children which did eat the portion of the king's meat."*

But Daniel's fairer and fatter flesh was the result of eating in *faith,* because his trust was in God. If eating vegetables and water were a health secret revealed in Scripture, then Jesus would have eaten only vegetables and water. We know that He did not.

What About Sweets?

Perhaps more than any food today, we read about sugar and sweets. Overweight people have long looked upon sweets as forbidden fruit. What about sweets? Does Scripture teach that it is wrong

101

to eat sweets? Are they the "deceitful meats" spoken of in Proverbs?

Actually, Scripture is filled with references to sweets, and there is a consistent pattern. When God spoke of the Promised Land, He called it a land *"that floweth with milk and honey"* (Leviticus 20:24). Again in Deuteronomy 8:8, God said He would lead them into a good land, a land of *"wheat, and barley, and vines, and fig trees, and pomegranates; a land of oil olive and honey."*

When reading these Scriptures, keep in mind that honey is even sweeter than sugar. Honey has 64 calories to a tablespoon and sugar only has 46. Even syrups do not duplicate the sweetness of honey.

We are told that God led Moses through the wilderness, and *"he instructed him, he kept him as the apple of his eye"* (Deuteronomy 32:10). And what did He do for this man He kept as the apple of His eye? *"He made him ride on the high places of the earth, that he might eat the increase of the fields; and he made him to suck honey out of the rock"* (Deuteronomy 32:13). God felt sweets were important enough that He performed a miracle in order to provide honey for Moses. We are told he ate the increase of the fields, so obviously, other food was available. Yet, God provided *honey!*

Honey's Value

Some of the highest words of praise in Scripture

have to do with sweetness. Ezekiel described the Word of God in Ezekiel 3:3 saying, *"It was in my mouth as honey for sweetness."* In Psalm 19:7, David extols God with magnificent praises saying, *"The law of the Lord is perfect, converting the soul: the testimony of the Lord is sure, making wise the simple."* He sums up with, *"more to be desired are they than gold, yea, than much fine gold: sweeter than honey and the honeycomb."* Would David or Ezekiel compare the Word of God to something that was sinful or bad for us?

God's great prophet, Isaiah, prophesied, *"The Lord himself shall give you a sign; behold, a virgin shall conceive, and bear a son, and shall call his name Immanuel"* (Isaiah 7:14). We have all read this with joy! It foretells the birth of our Lord. The next verse says, *"Butter and honey shall he eat"* (Isaiah 7:15). We know He actually ate honey because in Luke 24:42, when He asked for food from the disciples, *"They gave him a piece of broiled fish, and of an honeycomb. And he took it, and did eat before them."* Again, Jesus ate exactly as He instructed His disciples. He ate whatever was set before Him.

In all of Scripture, there is not a single instance where sweetness is used to mean anything but goodness. These are only a few of many examples. In fact, Proverbs 24:13 couldn't be any plainer. *"Eat thou honey, because it is good; and the honeycomb, which is sweet to thy taste."* It is supposed to taste good. God went to a lot of trouble making you able to taste sweets.

Living In Moderation

In Proverbs we are told to eat honey (sweets) because it is good and sweet to our taste. We are also cautioned that, *"It is not good to eat much honey."* (Proverbs 25:16). Scripture says, *"Hast thou found honey? Eat so much as is sufficient for thee."* (Proverbs 25:27,16). Paul tells us in Philippians 4:5 to, *"Let your moderation be known unto all men."*

What does that mean for us today? It means it is all right to eat sweets. God meant for you to enjoy them, but eat only as much as is *"sufficient for thee."* If you buy a package of six little doughnuts, and, after eating two or three, you are filled, don't eat the whole package. Moderation means that if half of a candy bar is sufficient for you, don't eat all of it!

Often just a taste is enough. During the time my husband lost his forty-five pounds, he occasionally took doughnuts for the workers in his office. He said he was amazed to find that sometimes one-forth of a doughnut was enough to satisfy him. Sometimes a taste is not enough to satisfy us. But learn to eat only *"so much as is sufficient for thee."* Don't eat what everyone else is eating, or how much is in the package, but how much is sufficient for *you*.

True Deceitful Meats

Deceitful meats then are not sweets, rather they are foods eaten for the wrong reasons, because of frustration, guilt, anger, or boredom. They are foods eaten to help you forget your troubles rather than turn to God.

Some people have used sweets as "deceitful meats." They have experienced an unnatural, obsessive, craving for sweets. They have eaten sweets to their condemnation so many times they think sweets are sinful. It was the gluttonous eating of sweets that was wrong, not the sweets themselves.

If a person has a problem with lust and reads sensual books, that is wrong. But reading isn't wrong, and books aren't wrong. Being able to read is a gift from God, but it can be used the wrong way. So it is that we can use foods the wrong way without the food itself being wrong.

We have looked at sugar, or honey, from a scriptural standpoint because that is the view that will stand. Even in the medical community there is no agreement about sugar being bad. I quote from the column, "Medical Q & A," a medical column carried in newspapers all over the country and written by Dr. Neil Solomon.

Medical View Of Sugar

A gentleman had written in because his wife was

trying to get him to stop using sugar. He asked Dr. Solomon:

"If I am wrong about the use of sugar, in what is an otherwise sound diet, I'd like to be told about it."

Here are some excerpts from his reply,

"I can say *there is little to suggest* that the use of sugar contributes significantly to cardiovascular disease, diabetes, or surprisingly, obesity." (It should not surprise us since God's Word says sweets are all right, but obesity is not.)

He goes on to cite a study by Dr. Frank Nuttall which showed, "Even though sugar consumption in the United States has either remained the same or increased slightly since 1968, deaths from coronary heart disease have decreased. Similarly, death from coronary heart disease is low in Cuba, Venezuela, and Colombia, even though sugar consumption in these countries is very high.

"As for development of diabetes, the primary determining factor in the case of adults is *obesity, not sugar consumption.*"

Direction For Today

What we are seeing today is a fulfillment of the prophecy given by Paul in 1 Timothy 4:1-4, *"Now the Spirit speaketh expressly, that in the latter times* (we know we are in the latter times) *some shall depart from the faith, giving heed to seducing spirits, and doctrines of devils. . .forbidding to marry and commanding to abstain from meats* (that is foods) *which God hath created to be received with thanksgiving of them which believe and know the truth. For every creature of God is good and nothing to be refused, if it be received with thanksgiving.*"

These two teachings *did* arise in exactly the same time frame, just as Paul predicted. The idea of living together instead of getting married surfaced at almost the exact time as the "wrong to eat sugar, wrong to eat meats" teachings.

He goes on to say, *"If thou put the brethren in remembrance of these things, thou shalt be a good minister of Jesus Christ"* (1 Timothy 4:6). So let me say it again—*food is not sinful—overeating is.* It is not wrong to eat meat; it is not wrong to eat sugar; it is not wrong to eat non-organic foods, it is not wrong to eat processed foods.

Conversely, it is not holy to eat organic foods. It is not holy to abstain from sugar. It is not holy to abstain from meat.

Natural Desires For Healthful Foods

This is not to say that nutrition has no place in our lives, but we are not to build our lives around it. As a person begins to eat from real hunger, he has a natural desire for more healthful foods.

To illustrate this, picture yourself on a camping trip. One day you decide to climb a big hill by the camp area. You begin early, and it takes a long time to get to the top. Every once in a while you stop to rest, and then you continue your climb. It is a beautiful, clear day. At the top, the view is breathtaking, and you spend quite a while admiring the view.

As you start down the hill, it is evening and you realize you haven't eaten all day. When you finally get back to camp, you are really hungry. On one side are cookies, candy bars, and potato chips. On the other side is a pan with fresh fish frying, corn on the cob, and maybe some fresh tomatoes. Which foods would you choose? Of course, the universal response is to choose the fish, corn, etc.

We do this exercise in class to illustrate our *natural desire* for more healthful foods when we eat only from real hunger. It is all part of the perfect God-given hunger response.

Deprived Childhood

Dr. William Slonecker, the well-known pediatrician from Nashville, Tennessee, had this to say about children who have eating problems. "The problem is that we do not let that child get hungry. Any child that has never been hungry, I feel, is a deprived child. He needs to be hungry enough to know what good, solid food tastes like."

My youngest daughter has a friend who has eaten nothing but "health foods" all her life. She never even tasted a cookie until she was three years old. That was because she ate one at nursery school. Her mother drives all over town to find organic foods. They never use sugar.

They do everything "right" as far as nutrition is concerned, but that child is always sick! She is always getting a cold, fever, or whatever is going around. My daughter is almost never sick, and we eat all things in moderation. Sickness comes from Satan and "the weapons of our warfare are not carnal, but mighty through God" (2 Corinthians 10:4).

Your Source Of Strength

Our strength and our health comes from God. We are told in Isaiah 40:31, *"They that wait upon the Lord shall renew their strength; they shall mount up with wings as eagles; They shall run and not be weary; and they shall walk and not faint."*

Paul tells us in 1 Timothy 4:8, *"Bodily exercise profiteth little: but godliness is profitable unto all things."* Godliness is profitable to our bodies! Proverbs doesn't tell us, "Attend to your diet, let not concern about what you eat depart from thine eyes for it is health to all your flesh." Rather it says, *"My son attend to my words; incline thine ear unto my sayings. Let them* (God's Words) *not depart from thine eyes; keep them* (God's Words) *in the midst of thine heart. For they* (God's Words) *are life unto those that find them, and health to all their flesh"* (Proverbs 4:20,21).

I have seen people who are just as obsessed with *what* they eat as gluttons are about *how much* they eat. Some of the most ungodly people I know eat nothing but health foods and exercise constantly. Their *body* has become their top priority.

There are also some very godly people who eat nothing but health foods, and that is fine. The point is that it doesn't matter what you eat as long as food and eating keep their proper place in your life.

Why Is This Freedom Important To Know?

It is important to have this freedom with regard to what we eat. If you think certain foods are sinful, Satan will heap condemnation upon you each time you eat them. If you eat a candy bar, he will say, "Well you know you shouldn't have eaten that. Now you have blown it. You might as well go ahead and gorge now." Condemnation over eating that one candy bar will cause you to eat three other candy bars, two doughnuts, and all of the last night's leftovers!

Conversely, when you see from God's Word that it is not wrong to eat that candy bar, but that you should only eat *"so much as is sufficient for thee"* (Proverbs 25:16), you will begin to eat smaller portions of a big candy bar. Without condemnation over eating a chocolate, you will begin to eat one or two instead of half the box. You will begin to cut yourself small pieces of pie because you will no longer feel you must "eat, drink, and be merry" because tomorrow you may diet. Rather, you will know that if you want more tomorrow, it will be all right to eat more.

Freedom In Action

I recently saw this principle beautifully illustrated. I was having lunch with a woman who lost over fifty pounds through Scriptural Eating Patterns. We had a lovely lunch, and afterward the waiter brought us an elegant dessert menu. The menu listed crepes filled with whipped cream and covered with fresh strawberries or a special praline sauce. We both felt totally free to order any dessert on the menu. But we had already eaten "so much as (was) sufficient for (us)." We decided not to eat dessert.

We made this choice in total freedom. It was different than when we were compulsive eaters. If we had ordered the dessert before we had been healed, we would have felt tremendous condemnation. Guilt would have led us to continue eating all day because we "already blew it for today."

If we had *not* ordered the dessert, but still wanted it, we would have thought about that dessert for the rest of the day. We might have even eaten other foods trying to satisfy that desire. Being free to eat all things, it was a simple decision. There would have been no condemnation if we had ordered it, and there was no lingering desire when we did not. *That's freedom, and it's wonderful*.

Why Are You Eating?

It is not *what* you eat but *why* you eat that is

important to God. You can sinfully overeat carrot sticks. You can sinfully overeat celery. You can sinfully overeat any food. In Psalm 78:27-31, we see this illustrated. *"He rained flesh also upon them as dust, and feathered fowls like as the sand of the sea."*

Now there was certainly nothing wrong with the quails since God Himself provided them. But as we read on, we are told, *"So they did eat, and were well filled:* (not "filled" but "well filled") *for he gave them their own desire; They were not estranged from their lust* (for food). *But while their meat was yet in their mouths, The wrath of God came upon them, and smote down the chosen men of Israel."* It was not what they ate, but why they ate.

Romans 14:20 says, *"All things indeed are pure; but it is evil for that man who eateth with offense."* If after reading these Scriptures you do not have total freedom to eat all things yet, *don't eat them.* Scripture says, *"For one believeth that he may eat all things: another, who is weak, eateth herbs. Let not him that eateth despise him that eateth not; and let not him which eateth not judge him that eateth "* (Romans 14:2,3). I believe that as you study God's Word you will come to have this freedom. But until you do, don't go against your conscience.

Convictions About Food

Some people feel a conviction that they

shouldn't eat certain foods. I once heard Oral Roberts tell about a very precious friend who didn't eat pork. When they ate together, his friend merely said, "Brother Oral, I feel a conviction that I should not have pork."

Oral respected this, although he felt no such conviction. Neither tried to persuade the other of the "error of their thinking," but lived the Scripture, *"Let not him which eateth not judge him that eateth."*

God never desires that individual convictions about food or drink divide His body. The question is, "Who is Lord of your life?"

Jesus reminds us in Matthew 11:18,19, *"For John came neither eating nor drinking, and they say, He hath a devil. The Son of man came eating and drinking, and they say, Behold a man gluttonous, and a winebibber."* At one point Jesus said, *"Among them that are born of women there hath not risen a greater than John the Baptist"* (Matthew 11:11). Yet He ate exactly the opposite of John.

During the time of my healing, there were certain foods which I knew I consistently tended to overeat. I avoided these foods as seed to the Spirit and as a way of choosing God in my eating. Now I can eat all foods with complete freedom. But start where you are.

People can get so caught up in eating or not eating certain foods that they miss the whole point—*Jesus is the answer*—not what foods we eat or don't eat. Our body is not sanctified by the food we eat, but rather our food is sanctified by the Word of God and prayer. (See 1 Timothy 4:5.)

Chapter 8

GIVING THANKS

When we think of saying grace before we eat, we often have a mental picture of a Norman Rockwell type family. They are sitting around the table at Sunday dinner, heads bowed and eyes closed. The children are peeking or secretly feeding the dog their brussel sprouts. Sweet and serene families gathered together.

But when Jesus gave thanks to God for His food, things happened! When He thanked God for the five loaves and two fishes, they were multiplied to feed over five thousand men, women, and children with twelve baskets of food left over! *"(He) took the five loaves, and the two fishes, and looking up to heaven, he blessed, and brake, and gave the loaves to his disciples, and the disciples to the multitude. And they did all eat"* (Matthew 14:19,20). Again in Matthew 15:36 we read that as Jesus took the seven loaves and fishes and gave thanks, they were multiplied to feed four thousand men, plus women and children. *"And he took the seven loaves and the fishes, and gave thanks, and brake them, and gave to his disciples, and the disciples to the multitude. And they did all eat.''* It was at the precise moment when Jesus blessed the bread that the disciples' eyes were opened to know Him. *"And it came to pass, as he sat at meat with them, he took bread, and blessed it, and brake, and gave to them. And their eyes were opened, and they knew him; and he vanished out of their sight"* (Luke 24:30,31).

Releasing Supernatural Power

There was a release of supernatural power when Jesus thanked God for His food. Paul tells us in 1 Timothy 4:4,5, *"nothing (is) to be refused, if it be received with thanksgiving: For it is sanctified by the word of God and prayer.''* Sanctified means purified, made conducive to spiritual blessing, freed from sin.

While Jesus placed little emphasis on *what* He ate, He placed great emphasis on *praying* over His food, thanking God for what He was about to eat. One of the things we teach in our Scriptural Eating Classes is the importance of thanking God for our food. A person who is seeking victory with their eating should thank God every time they begin to eat anything.

Least Likely To Say Grace

Have you ever noticed how often a person thanks God for their food on a binge? *Never!* When a person is alone, that is the time they are the *least* likely to thank God for their food and ask His blessing on it. But that is the most important time.

When we head to the kitchen for a "little snack," that is the time we are the least likely to say grace over our food. Yet, that is the time we are most likely to eat to our condemnation—to sinfully overeat.

During the time of my healing, God led me to pray over everything I ate. I don't mean that I prayed over each bite of food during a meal, but I do mean that I prayed over *every time* I started to eat. I still remember the prayer after all these years. "Father, I pray that You will bless this food to the strength and nourishment of my body, that it might not serve as condemnation, that I might not hate others or myself."

Praying before you eat is especially important when you are alone. Often just the act of thanking God for the food you are about to eat is enough to stop you from eating it. It is impossible to sincerely thank God for food you know you should not be eating. *I have never known a glutton who consistently prayed over everything they ate.*

Praying Before Temptation Arrives

Peter learned a bitter lesson about the power of prayer *before* you enter into temptation. Jesus prayed the night before He was betrayed. He told Peter he would deny Him, but Peter was full of confidence. *"Though all men shall be offended*

because of thee, yet will I never be offended"
(Matthew 26:33). Peter meant this with all his
heart as he was saying it.

Later, as Jesus prepared Himself for His coming
trial through prayer, Peter fell asleep. Jesus woke
Peter and told him to, *"Watch and pray, that ye
enter not into temptation; the spirit indeed is
willing but the flesh is weak"*(Matthew 26:41).
Jesus was telling Peter that if he would take the
time to prepare himself spiritually through prayer,
he would not have to give in to the temptation that
would later break Peter's heart. Conversely, Jesus
was warning him that if he did not pray, he would
enter into temptation and fall because the flesh is
weak. His good intentions were not enough to see
him through this temptation.

Strengthening Your Good Intentions

I see so much correlation between this episode
and people caught in any compulsive sin. How
many times they go to sleep confident that
"tomorrow I am going to do better." Like Peter,
we all have good intentions. We mean it with all
our heart. We don't intend to fall, but we are still
trusting in our flesh which is weak.

The Bible says that Peter wept bitterly. He was
angry with himself and full of condemnation. He
cried bitter tears of regret. This is a familiar pattern to a person caught in compulsive sin. Jesus
said Peter could have been spared this temptation

if he had taken the time to prepare himself through prayer, *beforehand.*

"Watch and pray that ye enter not into temptation." Watch—be alert to the danger. Plan out your day with non-eating activities. And pray—pray before you enter into temptation. Peter's prayers would have made the difference for him, and your prayers will make the difference in your being able to stand.

Chapter 9

A PLAN TO LAST A LIFETIME

Now that I have been free from compulsive eating (gluttony) for over ten years, I still observe the two-meal-a-day eating pattern four or five days a week. I think this eating pattern is one of the reasons my healing has been complete and will last for the rest of my life. It is a better way of eating, and I will never go back to three meals a day.

I do, however, allow myself more freedom to eat snacks. I don't hesitate to eat an ice cream cone with the kids or coffee cake with a friend. It is a beautiful thing to be able to eat these things without condemnation, to know it will not bring on a binge. I thank God for freedom from that nagging urge to eat.

I also have lunch when a friend invites me. If I have a luncheon meeting, I go, eat lunch, and thoroughly enjoy it! There is certainly no condemnation when I eat lunch. I just don't eat three meals a day on a consistent basis.

Hunger By Suggestion

I have found that if I know I am going to be eating lunch, I will actually be hungry by lunchtime. Whereas, if I know I am not going to eat lunch that day, I will not be hungry. That is why it is important to *purpose in your heart* when you are going to observe the lunch fast or dinner fast. Simply tell your body when you wake up that morning, this is how it is going to be!

One of the reasons I feel this has been such a satisfactory plan for all these years—and will continue to be for the rest of my life—is that *I never give up the foods I enjoy when I eat.* Again, let me repeat that dieting is not mentioned in Scripture, but fasting is. For we are *"dead with Christ from the rudiments of the world* (and commandments and doctrines of men which say) *touch not, taste not: handle not; which are all to perish with the using. . . .* (But rather we) *set* (our) *affections* (focus of our life) *on things above, not on things on the earth* (constant concern about what we are going to eat, when we are going to eat, how much we are going to eat)" (Colossians 2:20; 3:2).

Man Lives By The Word of God

We have some precious friends who are going to Mexico as missionaries, and *what* they are going to eat is the furthest thing from their minds and hearts. They are going to loose God's Word to lost people. They have *"set* (their) *affection on things above."* God is their Source.

When Jesus had fasted for forty days and forty nights, Satan came to tempt Him with food saying, *"If thou be the Son of God, command this stone that it be made bread"* (Luke 4:3). Today he says, "You can't go without food! You'll ruin your health. Think of your protein! Think of your vitamins!"

"But Jesus answered him, saying, *It is written, That man shall not live by bread alone, but by every word of God"* (Luke 4:4).

God's Word is the answer. We see in later Scriptures where Jesus ate and enjoyed His food. He ate as He instructed His disciples, *"such things as are set before you,"* but His priorities were right.

To lose weight *you must not eat at all between meals.* To maintain your weight you may have snacks from time to time. You may always have things to drink, and not only diet drinks. If you are really hungry (not bored, frustrated, or feeling guilty) a glass of juice, hot tea with sugar, or hot chocolate will curb your hunger.

It doesn't take much to curb real hunger. It is also worth noting that real hunger pains do not last all day. They only last about thirty minutes. Try timing them the next time you fast.

It is all right to have something to drink—*just don't start eating.* You must break the pattern of eating. As you retrain your body, you will be hungry to start with. People who have been overeating for a long time can experience some weakness. *This is not real hunger, but rather withdrawal symptoms.*

It will become easier and easier, and hunger will come less and less. It will become easier to draw your attention away from food. Each time you sow to the Spirit, you have overcome the flesh (overeating) a little bit more.

Some Benefits Of Eating Two Meals

I have found that if I have gained a few extra pounds on vacation or over a holiday (and you will from time to time), I actually look forward to getting back to a schedule of two meals a day. I miss being hungry when I eat! Almost everyone has, at some time, experienced a time when they were not able to eat and were quite hungry when they finally ate.

The food just seemed to taste extra good. I have had similar comments from others who have tried eating only two meals a day. They are amazed at how easily their bodies adapt, and how good their food tastes.

If you are in the weight losing phase, and you are not losing as fast as you would like, cut back some on the amount you eat for both of your meals. It's *easy* to kid yourself about how much you're eating, but the scales won't lie! *Do not start restricting what you eat, only how much you eat.* Don't get back in the "lettuce and tomato" syndrome. Go ahead and eat the foods you enjoy, but eat somewhat less until you find the amount you can eat and still lose weight.

Lifetime Habits

Remember, we are talking about a lifetime change in your eating habits. If you restrict yourself from the foods you enjoy, you will not want to cut back on your eating after a holiday for example. Just be *faithful* with the fasting you offer to God. It's fine to start small, just be sure you start faithful. *"He that is faithful in that which is least is faithful also in much"* (Luke 16:10). Be faithful in your daily fasting, and you will be faithful also in the larger things (weight loss).

Adoptable Plan For Business

My husband, Don, has recently lost over 45 pounds eating this way. So, I asked him to give a testimony to our class. Don was not a compulsive eater, he was one of those people who was overweight and said, "It doesn't really matter."

He shared with us that although he had seen the victory in my life for the last ten years and knew what a wonderful change it made, he hadn't tried eating only two meals a day. As he reviewed the class materials with me, especially proofreading this book, he said he found that it *did* matter! He had a real desire to lose his extra weight by sowing to the Spirit rather than to the flesh.

However, he found that skipping lunch didn't work with his lifestyle. He owns a consulting engineering firm, and sometimes he must take clients out to lunch. Other times he simply needs a break from his concentration and really looks forward to lunch. As a result, he used the same principles but skipped dinner instead. He found it was not difficult for him to skip dinner several nights as seed to the Spirit.

He lost seventeen pounds the first five weeks. The best part is that he is keeping the weight off, and his body is beginning to respond to his God-given hungry and full responses. We recently had a weekend with quite a bit of entertaining. By Sunday we were both saying how we couldn't wait to get back to two meals!

Changing Attitude

Don tried many diets before, only to regain the weight he lost as he returned to his normal eating pattern. This time his whole attitude about food is changing. His appetite is also coming in line with his God-given hungry and full responses. That is why it will last.

He has also noticed the extra time added to his week nights! The men and women in my class wanted to know how this could work out with the family. They wondered about my skipping lunch and his skipping dinner several nights a week.

More Time To Enjoy

When Don is not going to eat dinner with us, he calls to let me know ahead of time. I feed the girls and myself early, which is fine with us since we are all hungry early. By the time he arrives, the kitchen is clean, the girls are fed, and we can sit, talk, and relax together. If we need to go somewhere that evening, we have extra time to get ready. If the girls need help with their school work, we have at least an extra hour.

Does this mean I don't think families should eat together? No, No, and No! It only means that our family life is not built around eating together. If we eat together, it is good. If we don't eat together, it is good. Just because we don't eat together does not mean we can't be together doing something else. Which is better? Eating together or walking together? Together is together.

So as Paul said in Romans 14:6, *"He that eateth, eateth to the Lord, for he giveth God thanks; and he that eateth not, to the Lord he eateth not, and giveth God thanks."*

I have found victory in many other areas of my life by using God's Word and sowing to the Spirit rather than to the flesh. My healing from gluttony was the beginning of my realization of Who Jesus is, and what He really did for us. I will always have a special place in my heart for overweight people because I have been there. I know what it feels like inside. But now I am thin, and I know what that feels like, too. I thank God for the freedom which He purchased for us through His own Son, Jesus.

Chapter 10

SEVEN ROADBLOCKS TO
TOTAL HEALING

I have seen people in our classes begin in great victory. Their faces glow with spiritual illumination, but occasionally it begins to fade. I have found there are seven areas where it is easy to fall. If you are not experiencing all the success you feel you should be, check yourself in these seven areas:

1. *Trying to take on the whole problem at once instead of taking one day at a time as Jesus instructed.* (See Matthew 6:34.) We are given the grace, the strength, and the power to live in total victory this day. Don't try to take on the whole problem at once. One woman shared that for over a month after coming to class, she had no weight loss. She said that each week after class she would think, "Tomorrow I am going to fast for two or three days." And each week she would not even make it home without eating. The next week she

would again get stirred up and decide, "Tomorrow I am really going to fast.

Finally, she decided to only take that day. She resolved in her heart to be faithful until she got home after class. The next day, she determined not to eat between meals, and to offer the fasting to God. Before long, she was fasting one entire meal and losing weight. This change came because she started by taking one day at a time.

2. *Getting back into the "diet syndrome," restricting yourself from certain foods.* The "diet syndrome" says, "I've already had pancakes for breakfast.I might as well eat today." A woman called to ask for prayer. I prayed with her and suggested that she determine in her heart what seed she was going to sow to the Spirit when we hung up the phone. She said, "I've already eaten some candy—I guess I'll have to wait until tomorrow." Since this is not a diet, you have never blown it for the day! *"A just man falleth seven times and riseth up again."* (Proverbs 24:16). Simply rise up again! Start sowing to the Spirit from that moment.

3. *Knowingly sowing to the flesh.* (See Galatians 6:7 and Romans 6:16.) Before you read this book, you may not have realized there were certain times and activities when you consistently tended to overeat. Each time you now choose this activity, you are sowing to the flesh. If you continue to sow to the flesh, you will continue to reap

from the flesh. Resist the devil. Move into "non-eating" activities.

4. *Leaving your house empty.* (See Matthew 12:43.) Jesus tells us that when the unclean spirit is gone out of a man (the spirit of overeating) that it looks for another place to live. But if it can't find one it returns. If the house is empty (still watching TV), it brings seven other spirits more wicked than itself (Mr. Binge, Mr. Condemnation, Mr. Depression). You cannot stand on God's Word without a foundation. Don't leave your house empty—fill yourself with God's Word. You can't stand on God's Word if you don't *know* God's Word. Find Scriptures to help you not to worry or feel other negative emotions.

5. *Sowing from your abundance rather than from your want.* (See Mark 12:44.) What was sowing from your want last week may not be sowing from your want this week. You know when you are sowing from your want, and God knows when you are sowing from your want. Sowing from your want is not skipping a meal that you normally skip. It is not working through your lunch hour when the boss tells you to work through your lunch hour. *Sowing from your want is what you give up for His (Jesus') sake and the gospel's.* (See Mark 10:29.)

6. *Sowing in a hit or miss manner.* (See 2 Corinthians 9:6.) We are told in this passage that he who *"soweth sparingly shall also reap sparingly."* If you sow to the Spirit one day and not the

next, fast on Monday and eat Tuesday through Thursday, then maybe try fasting on Friday, you will reap the same kind of help. If you sow sparingly (hit-or-miss commitment), you will also reap sparingly (hit-or-miss help).

7. *Not being faithful with the seed you have decided to sow.* (See Luke 16:10.) Don't take on more than you can handle. Start where you are. Don't be afraid to start small—but start faithfully. Humanly we want to start big, but Jesus said to start small. In Matthew 13:31, He compared the Kingdom of heaven to a tiny mustard seed. *"The kingdom of heaven* (with regard to gluttony) *is like to a grain of mustard seed,* (small seeds sown to the Spirit from your want), *which a man took, and sowed in his field* (your life): **Which indeed is the greatest among herbs** (biggest problem in your life taken care of), *and becometh a tree, so that the birds of the air come and lodge in the branches thereof* (you will be a witness and blessing to others with the same problem)."

You don't have to ask yourself, "Is this going to work?" God's Word works 100% of the time. You can be free for the rest of your life in Jesus' name.

That freedom is what Jesus Christ, the Savior of the world, the sacrificial lamb, the Son of Man, is all about.

Chapter 11

A MAN'S PERSPECTIVE
by Don Hampton

I had spent my entire life, thirty-seven years, being basically overweight. Not always fat, but never slim. I began battling hypertension, or high blood pressure, at the age of fifteen. I never really attempted to maintain my weight. I was active and always tall for my age.

In my younger years I thought I was ten or fifteen pounds overweight. In reality, the scales showed I was over twenty pounds too heavy. As the years crept by, and my life style became more sedentary, the scales began creeping constantly upward.

The gain was consistent but slow. I would occasionally try one of Diane's many new "fad" diets. YUK! I still remember the banana and milk diet. I didn't care much for bananas to begin with. That was almost twenty years ago, and I still cringe when I pass a bunch of bananas in the store.

Naturally, none of the diets had a lasting effect. I

still preferred my double serving of chili, hot dogs, or Mexican food. Sometime in my early thirty's, I unconsciously decided not to actively fight my weight anymore. Life was easier at that point because the frustration caused by dieting was gone. But the excess weight continued to silently do its deadly damage. My weight rose from 220 to 230, 235, and finally to over 240 pounds.

Kidding Myself

Boy, was I oblivious to my own surroundings! Diane's weight was well under control. She hadn't been on any silly diets for eight or ten years. She was much happier. I didn't find her crying about her weight anymore. She really looked super and had looked great for years.

She had talked about how God healed her of compulsive eating, and I thought, "Great!" But, it didn't make much sense to me. Besides, I didn't look so bad at 240 pounds! Since my awakening, it amazes me how overweight people deceive themselves.

After having maintained her weight for ten years, Diane had an opportunity to share her experience. We expected a small group of about half a dozen ladies. That group of six was closer to fifty, and grew to over one hundred men and women. The group continued to meet for about nine months! Sometimes Diane taught three different classes each week. People were hungry to hear what God could do in this area.

After our pastor reviewed the class materials, he asked Diane if she had ever considered writing a book. Diane also felt the class needed something written to enable them to better grasp these concepts. Also, she was receiving many invitations to speak, and she was physically unable to meet all the demands herself. With my encouragement, she began writing. This was the birth of Scriptural Living Ministries and Diane's first book. You are reading an expanded version of the original book, *Scriptural Eating Patterns*.

A Witness To His Wonders

As a faithful and loving husband, I began proofreading and critiquing each page. I am positive that I must have read the original book at least thirty-two times before we decided it was ready to print. Let me tell you this, after reading a book thirty-two times, you *know* what the book is about! I decided, along with a little encouragement from the Lord, that maybe I wasn't a very good witness being overweight.

I began putting God's principles about weight and eating to use in my life. I immediately discovered that following them exactly as set forth in the book did not fit my schedule as a businessman. I often spent the lunch hour with clients. I wasn't going to tell my client, "I am fasting, but go ahead and enjoy a nice meal." No way. Still, the principles made sense to me.

Being quick to learn (after all, it only took me eleven years and thirty-two times through the book to figure out why Diane remains slim and trim) I made a slight modification to the program. Breakfast was out. I ate a normal, enjoyable lunch, and, for most of the next three months, I skipped dinner.

I never stopped eating the foods I enjoyed. I still ate chili and Mexican food, but I considered my full response. I ordered only one double chili burger instead of two. I even got to the point where I didn't even order a double. The whole program fit in well with my schedule as a businessman.

Three months, forty-five pounds, and six inches off the waist later, I was amazed to see that the excess weight was gone forever. That was almost five years ago. A couple of years later, during a period of heavy stress, I began to let go of the principles and I gained weight. I reapplied God's Word, however, and my body came right back into subjection to me.

Blood Pressure Miracle

Two amazing—really miraculous—things occurred as I applied God's Word. Of course, I lost weight, but my high blood pressure (essential hypertension, which is considered incurable) began to drop into the normal range. The first time in twenty years! The doctor had no explanation for this. So, I gave him one of Diane's books. I give the glory to God. Diets never affected my blood pressure, but the principles in God's Word did.

The second thing is that for the first time in my life, I am not under bondage to eat at a certain time. Before, if I was even late for a meal, I was shaky, sick, and irritable. Believe me, I *never* missed a meal! Now I can go all day without eating if necessary. Sometimes I get into a business meeting where we need to work through the lunch hour. Now, it is no problem for me.

Not Always Easy

Sometimes I teach the last class of a series, and I always point out that the weight loss period was *not* always easy for me. There were times when I was hungry. I was surprised to find that this hunger was often more easily satisfied than I ever dreamed possible.

Sometimes doughnuts or fresh cookies would show up at the office. The temptation for a taste would really get to me. I defeated this by saying, "OK taste buds, you want a taste? That's all you are going to have." That one taste was enough for me, and it satisfied that driving urge to eat. Eventually, I was able to bypass even that small sample.

I praise God and thank Him for raising up Diane to teach Scriptural Eating Patterns. I know that through a healthier body, God has given me a new lease on life. As you complete this book, my prayers are with you. I pray that you will have the courage to make a commitment that will enable God to give *you* a new lease on life.

COMMONLY ASKED QUESTIONS:

Question: I am a diabetic. What about me?

Answer: In every situation, there is always a way to sow to the Spirit. Obviously, you did not become overweight by following the diabetic diet. Look at the times you have the most problems with eating and begin sowing those times to the Spirit. Also, you could simply purpose in your heart to follow the diet your doctor gave you. Offer that to God as seed to the Spirit. *Do what you can do and God will do what you cannot do.*

Question: Is it safe to eat two meals when you are pregnant?

Answer: Yes! First, let's look at your question scripturally. God Himself would feed His creation correctly. Therefore, we can see how He provided for pregnant women in Scripture.

In Exodus 16:12, we see the Lord providing for the children of Israel in the desert. He said, *"At even* (in the evening) *ye shall eat flesh, and in the morning ye shall be filled with bread.''* Two meals, morning and evening. We know, if we read further, that food was provided in such a way that it would be impossible to eat more often. In the morning, as the sun's heat increased, the food melted. If the Israelites tried to keep the manna overnight, it bred worms and began to stink.

We *know* that many of these women were pregnant because a whole generation was born in the wilderness. God made no special provision for the pregnant women. We can see that two meals a day is scripturally sound for pregnant women.

In my own experience, I had no trouble observing a two meal a day eating pattern during pregnancy. Although, I did drink a glass of milk or eat an occasional small snack if I felt hungry. As always, I found this eating pattern was a vital key to maintaining my weight. I gained exactly what the doctor suggested with both pregnancies. And I lost all the extra weight within a few months after giving birth. Both of our babies were fat and healthy—8 and 7½ pounds!

Question: When you are fasting, are drinks allowed?

Answer: Absolutely! The only exception would be if you have a real problem drinking too much. I drank coffee with cream, and one soda or a glass of fruit juice in the afternoon. But only if I desired it. Don't make fasting too hard on yourself! We are sowing *control* with our eating not a complete fast. We are looking for lifetime changes in our eating patterns. Total fasting could hardly become a lifetime eating pattern.

Question: How do you feel about diet foods?

Answer: For the most part, I believe it is a mistake to use diet products. They tend to promote the thinking, "It is *always* all right to eat this because it is low in calories;" or the idea, "I can eat all I want because it is low-calorie." You are not relearning your God-given hungry and full responses.

I also believe that diet foods have a much lower ability to satisfy. I never used any diet products during the time of my weight loss. It was a joy to be able to eat "real food" for the first time without condemnation. And, I found them much more satisfying.

Question: I have over one hundred pounds to lose. Will this work for me?

Answer: Yes and no. Yes, healing is available; and no, I do not feel that fasting one meal a day will meet your total need. The greatest success seems to come by cutting down to *one meal* a day. Almost every person who has had over one hundred pounds to lose has told me they find it just as easy to cut back to one meal.

Also, *increase your vegetable intake with your meal.* Many people with over one hundred pounds to lose don't eat any vegetables at all! This is far from the "moderation" which Scripture teaches. God can change your desire for certain foods!

Believe God for a change in the foods you really enjoy.

If your budget has been tight, and you have leaned toward starchy menus because of this, you will be able to afford meats you could not afford before. When you eliminate one or two meals a day, you will see quite a savings at the grocery store. One lady told me, "I was actually shocked to realize how much I was spending on food." One couple said they were able to afford steaks for the first time in their marriage! This doesn't mean you should cut out all starches. But avoid meals that use starches, such as macaroni and cheese, as a main dish. Eat all things but in moderation.

Question: I've had some real emotional upsets and a lot on my mind lately. Shouldn't I wait until things settle down before I try to deal with my eating?

Answer: Absolutely not! Emotional upsets and mental stress are greatly exaggerated and magnified by overeating. The Bible says, *"Bread eaten in secret is pleasant. . .but her guests are in the depths of hell"* (Proverbs 9:17,18). During such a time, you need something that is going to lift you up, not something that is going to drag you down to the depths of hell.

Time after time people report to me that as they bring their eating under control, the upsets seem to level out. They are better able to deal with the stress, they find new solutions to problems which seemed to overwhelm them. Every part of you—

body, mind, and spirit—functions more effectively when you are sowing to the Spirit.

Question: Couldn't this fasting lead to anorexia?

Answer: This has never been a problem with Scriptural Eating Patterns. The reason is simple: for the first time in their lives, people feel in *control* of their eating!

The word most often used when people describe the difference this teaching has made in their lives is *freedom.* People say, "I feel free for the first time in my life." "My whole life changed as I learned how to sow to the Spirit." A man recently wrote, "My attitude toward food has drastically altered, and my spirits seem to soar as my weight plummets." These are not thoughts and feelings which lead to anorexia.